Sustainable He

T0258595

Sustainable Health Care

Sustainable Healthcare

Knut Schroeder

General Practitioner (Family Physician), Concord Medical Centre
Honorary Senior Clinical Lecturer
Centre for Academic Primary Care
School of Social and Community Medicine
University of Bristol
Bristol, UK

Trevor Thompson

General Practitioner (Family Physician), Wellspring Healthy Living Centre
Reader in Healthcare Education
Centre for Academic Primary Care
School of Social and Community Medicine
University of Bristol
Bristol, UK

Kathleen Frith

President, Glynwood and former Managing Director
Center for Health and the Global Environment
Harvard Medical School
Boston, MA, USA

David Pencheon

Director
NHS Sustainable Development Unit
East of England Strategic Health Authority
Cambridge, UK

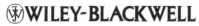

A John Wiley & Sons, Ltd., Publication

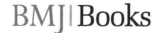

Library of Congress Cataloging-in-Publication Data
Sustainable healthcare / Knut Schroeder ... [et al.].

    p. ; cm.

Includes bibliographical references and index.

ISBN 978-0-470-65671-6 (pbk.)

I. Schroeder, Knut.

[DNLM: 1. Delivery of Health Care. 2. Climate Change. 3. Conservation of Natural Resources. W 84.1]

362.1 – dc23

2012030887

A catalogue record for this book is available from the British Library.

Wiley also publishes its books in a variety of electronic formats. Some content that appears in print may not be available in electronic books.

Cover design by: Rob Sawkins at Opta Design. Image adapted from iStock File #:5977539 © 2008 appleuzr

Set in 9.5/12pt Minion by Laserwords Private Limited, Chennai, India.

1   2013

Contents

Preface

Should people working in the health sector be interested in sustainability? The answer, we think, is a resounding 'yes'. We, an authorial team comprising a primary care clinician (KS), a medical teacher (TT), a public health specialist (DP) and a science educationalist (KF), have been exploring the interface between medicine and sustainability for many years. In that time, general public interest in this area has increased a lot, but within the health sector it has received relatively little attention. We have written this book as a synthesis of a growing, but disparate, body of expert knowledge, and also with the hope of bringing sustainability to its rightful place at the centre stage of healthcare policy and practice.

The earth system is a wonderful yet ultimately vulnerable thing. It provides us with endless benefits upon which we are entirely dependent and which we can easily come to take for granted. These 'ecosystems services' include fresh water, clean air, fertile soils, carbon-based and renewable energy sources and a stable and relatively predictable climate. Less tangibly, we draw spiritual sustenance from nature in all its beauty and diversity. The science is now unequivocal – this planetary system is under stress due to human activity. We unpack these stresses, such as climate change and the loss of biodiversity, and consider the various consequences for human health and the healthcare system – a system that itself struggles to contain costs, deal with the soaring prevalence of chronic illness and bring humanity to technological care.

This book describes a new paradigm to tackle these pressing predicaments – a collection of ideas and perspectives (mostly developed by others, but some of our own) that fall, however untidily, under the banner of *sustainable healthcare*. This brings to the foreground the prevention of disease and the creation of individual and community resilience. It champions lean systems of clinical care that maximise efficiency and common humanity and minimise resource use and the creation of waste products (including greenhouse gases and toxic pollutants). A consistent and heartening observation is that many interventions that improve individual health (such as fresh, local and mainly plant-based food) are also good for the health of the planetary system – creating what are termed 'virtuous cycles'.

We have written for a readership busy with the myriad tasks of delivering care. We have tried to keep the book concise and balance 'need to know' with 'useful to know' information. We have read and appraised much of the science so you don't have to, and tried to draw balanced conclusions in a field where there is considerable uncertainty. At times we have applied the *precautionary principle* – advocating action where the price of inaction seems incalculable. We cut through some of the jargon and challenge the rhetoric of both fear and denial, which often pervades the topic. And we focus on the essential questions, offering a synopsis of the main issues which we support with key references and links to sources of further information. In short, this is a book of first resort.

We write with a wide readership in mind including health professionals, educationalists, health service managers and healthcare students for whom it might provide an outline curriculum in sustainable healthcare. We hope this is a positive book that inspires reflection, engagement and – crucially – action. We think that there are smarter, safer, fairer and more sustainable ways of doing things in the health sector, which are well worth the effort for the benefit of current and future generations. Who would have thought even 10 years ago that in many countries smoking would be banned in public places? A similar shift in public policy and human behaviour, involving innovative technology and better models of care, needs to happen to develop health systems that can sustain us through the challenging decades ahead.

For feedback, comments and suggestions for improvements please email k.schroeder@bristol.ac.uk.

Knut Schroeder
General Practitioner (Family Physician), Concord Medical Centre;
Honorary Senior Clinical Lecturer, University of Bristol

Trevor Thompson
General Practitioner (Family Physician), Wellspring Healthy Living Centre;
Reader in Healthcare Education, University of Bristol

Kathleen Frith
President, Glynwood and former Managing Director, Center for Health and
the Global Environment, Harvard Medical School

David Pencheon
Director, NHS Sustainable Development Unit

Acknowledgements

We owe much gratitude to a number of people who helped tremendously with writing this book by providing us with key resources and materials and reading part or all of the manuscript. In alphabetical order, we are particularly grateful to:

Annie Anderson, Ari Bernstein, Stefi Barna, Jonathan Broad, Timmy Bouley, Peter Cawston, Adrian Davis, Bob Fox, Ian Fitzpatrick, Howard Frumkin, Lynn Gibbons, Michelle Gottlieb, Chris Johnstone, Phil Insall, Katy Mahood, Janet Maxwell, Frances Mortimer, Hubert Murray, Scott Murray, Chris Payne, David Peters, Ian Roberts, Katherine Rusack, Marion Steiner, Jerome Thomas, Ash Tierney, Sarah Walpole and Sarah Webster.

We would also like to thank Mary Banks, Adam Gilbert, Chrisma Ng, Jon Peacock, Sangeetha Parthasarathy and everyone else at Wiley for their patience, gentle guidance and their belief in this project. Many thanks also to Kevin Dunn for expert copy-editing.

We would also like to acknowledge the industry and dedication the many researchers, writers, clinicians and activists whose endeavours we have drawn on in the writing of this book.

About the authors

Knut Schroeder works part-time as a Family Physician and is Honorary Senior Clinical Lecturer at the Centre for Academic Primary Care in the University of Bristol, UK. He had never really considered the link between climate change and health until he attended a conference on *'Climate Change and its Impact on Health'* in 2008, hosted by the Royal College of Physicians. This instilled a growing interest in the relationship between health and sustainability and prompted the idea for writing this book. Knut is a Board Member of the UK *Self Care Forum*, which aims to support people in making better (as well as more sustainable) choices about their health. He also works with the *NHS Institute for Innovation and Improvement* to help family practices work more efficiently and more sustainably. Knut enjoys spending time with his young family. Whenever work and family commitments allow, he is out and about running or cycling, or writes about topics that he feels passionate about.

    Trevor Thompson is a Family Physician at the Wellspring Healthy Living Centre in Bristol, UK, which supports a diverse inner-city population with a range of community-based and medical services. He is also a senior teacher at the University of Bristol Medical School with responsibilities across the curriculum. Trevor has been reading on the theme of sustainability for many years and since 2006 has run an undergraduate course on the *'Global Environment and Human Health'*. Teaching is often the best way to learn and his writing here draws extensively on his educational practice which seeks to engage both hearts and minds. Trevor is clinical co-lead for the *Sustainable Healthcare Education Network*, supporting green educational initiatives across the UK. He is an active cyclist, sailor and grower.

    Kathleen Frith is a creative, visionary leader working for a smarter, more sustainable world and President of Glynwood, one of the United States' leading sustainable agriculture and food organisations. With a deep passion for the natural world, Kathleen studied marine biology and received a Master's degree in Science Journalism from Boston University. In 2001, she was recruited to Harvard by the *Center for Health and the Global Environment* at

Harvard Medical School, where she helped shape the Center's programmes to educate and inform people about the links between human health, the ocean, food systems and the environment, serving as the organisation's Managing Director during the last two years of her tenure. In 2009, Kathleen produced the award-winning film *Once Upon a Tide*, a live action and animated educational short that screens around the world. In 2010, Kathleen started the *Harvard Community Garden*, Harvard University's first garden dedicated solely to the production of food. Other initiatives while at the Center included the creation of the Center's *Healthy Oceans, Healthy HumansProgram*, the launch of Center's *Healthy and Sustainable Food Program* and work with National Geographic to help restore a healthy, sustainable seafood resource. Kathleen has produced a number of award-winning reports and publications and serves as an advisor for a number of environmental and community organisations.

David Pencheon is a UK-trained public health doctor and is currently Director of the National Health Service's *Sustainable Development Unit* for England. David was previously Director of a Public Health Observatory in Cambridge, England. He has worked as a clinical doctor in the NHS, a joint Director of Public Health, a Public Health Training Programme Director in the East of England, with the NHS R&D programme, and lived in China in the early 1990s contributing to the work of Save the Children Fund (UK). His main interests and areas of research and publication are: sustainable development, large scale transformational change, health and climate change, underpinning action and policy with good information and evidence, training and professional development, organisational development, medical informatics and decision support for health professionals, carers and the public. He blogs mainly via the BMJ website. He was awarded an OBE in the New Year's Honours List 2012 for services to public health and the NHS.

Chapter 1 **Greening the gaze**

Health professionals have a lot on their minds: caring for patients, managing teams, keeping up to date with clinical developments and responding to broader agendas of quality and cost containment. This book offers up a quietly revolutionary invitation to rethink this enterprise by considering medicine in its rightful place within a much bigger planetary system. Here, we call this new way of thinking *sustainable healthcare* and believe it can help us deliver services of better quality, at lower costs and with less impact on the systems that sustain us. To this point in time the health sector has taken planetary health for granted, but now a body of evidence shows an earth system under stress. Half the rainforest is gone, extinction rates are soaring, the oceans are increasingly acidic and the planet is running a fever one degree above pre-industrial levels. We are just starting to realise how these planetary ailments impact on human health, with climate change famously described in the *Lancet* as 'the biggest global health threat of the 21st century' [1]. Though many health professionals are alive to these global issues, in the health professions, as in society at large, sustainability competes with many other pressing and more proximate concerns. Thus, there is a danger that we are collectively sleepwalking into a public health catastrophe. This book offers a new synthesis of sustainability and health, leading in later chapters to many ideas for practical action. Firstly, though, we want to explain why we need a revolution in our health systems, why nothing short of a revolution is going to be enough and what sort of a revolution we are talking about. Luckily it is a revolution from which we all stand to benefit.

The revolutionary road

Nineteenth century medicine witnessed the emergence of *germ theory*, which revolutionised our understanding of infectious disease. This new theory dispatched the then prevalent *miasmatic* paradigm, which held that disease arose from bad air. In the twentieth century, classical mechanics was

Sustainable Healthcare, First Edition. Knut Schroeder, Trevor Thompson, Kathleen Frith and David Pencheon.

revolutionised by quantum theory, in which, for instance, matter could be both particulate and wave-like. Such paradigmatic revolution requires two conditions. Firstly, there needs to be a build-up of *anomalies*, difficulties that cannot be solved by the dominant paradigm and which call its completeness into question. Secondly, a new paradigm must be waiting in the wings that accounts for the problems of the day and offers some hope of resolving them. We argue that the time for such a paradigmatic revolution in medicine is upon us. Biomedicine, despite its huge successes, cannot, of itself, provide solutions to the long term health needs of humanity. So, what are these anomalies and predicaments that are great enough to signal the need for a revolutionary new approach?

The verge of collapse

Readers in New York or Glasgow or Sydney may be forgiven for thinking that it is business as usual in healthcare. People value medical care and hold healthcare professionals in high esteem, with the enterprise enjoying enduring governmental support. There are plenty of patients, plenty of things to do to help them and a reasonable amount of money available to pay for it all. In many ways, then, these readers are right. It takes a lot of imagination to think beyond our immediate circumstances, to think globally and think in terms of our common and distant future. Because while, as we shall see, there are challenges facing us right now, there are more and greater challenges ahead. The greatest would be the collapse of civil society through some sort of man-made environmental calamity, as in science fiction movies like *The Day After Tomorrow*. This possibility feels remote. It probably also felt remote to the many societies which have experienced such collapses in recorded history [2]. Take for instance the fate of the Easter Islands communities. These remote islands were first spotted on Easter Day 1722 by the Dutch explorer Jacob Roggeveen. He encountered a small population, with small and leaky canoes, living on an island devoid of trees, but sporting 300 stone platforms and 887 giant, long-eared, and intently gazing, stone statues. How, thought Roggeveen, did these Polynesians voyage in such vessels from their nearest neighbour, Pitcairn, 1300 miles away, and erect such monuments without rope and wood? Paleobotanical research has demonstrated that the islands were originally thickly wooded with a huge and now extinct species of palm. So what happened? We know that from around AD 900 settlers arrived and used trees for firewood, cremation, sea-worthy canoes and timber for shifting statues. They also cleared woodland to create fields to feed their workforce and a population of around 15 000. We know that by AD 1600 this complex tribal society had all but collapsed. All native land birds and mammals were extinct, all the trees gone and the stone quarries abandoned. The priestly caste was replaced by militia and the islanders turned to cannibalism. Of course, some people *survived* but by most reckonings in a much impoverished culture. Captain Cook visited the islands in 1774 and described the inhabitants as 'small, lean, timid and miserable'. The Easter Island story concerns a tiny geographical locale. But today we face the collapse of a planetary system that will affect us all.

Living within boundaries

When we look back on the Easter Islanders cutting down their trees and subverting their culture, we feel incredulous that people could be so short-sighted. But how will future generations look back on us? Will ours be branded the *Age of Stupid* [3]? Collapsing cultures consistently fail to play by the rules – rules that contemporary science is starting to name and understand. In 2009, the journal *Nature* published a feature based on the work of the *Stockholm Environment Institute* on *planetary boundaries* [4]. In a number of distinct domains, these boundaries define the estimated limits of what we can do without causing serious adverse changes to the planetary system (Table 1.1). The Institute proposes, for instance, a boundary for the loss of biodiversity of 'ten species lost to life per million species per year' and a boundary of 15% of global land cover converted to cropland (the current figure is 11.7%).

If we can keep within these boundaries, say the authors, we have a chance of maintaining the favourable earthly conditions of the *Holocene*. The Holocene is a geological epoch, beginning about 12 000 years ago, characterised by a stable interglacial climate. Geologists now speak informally of the *Anthropocene*, a new period which marks the time from which we can observe the impact of humanity on the global system: its oceans, soils, atmosphere, climate and biosphere (Chapter 2). The bottom line is not comforting. We are, through our activities, already approaching or surpassing all of the planetary boundaries cited by the Stockholm Institute. For instance, the authors of the article in *Nature* give a threshold of 350 parts per million (ppm) of atmospheric carbon dioxide to contain global warming at less than two degrees above pre-industrial levels. Yet, in February 2012, the official figure from Hawaii's Mauna Loa observatory put the figure at 394 ppm [5]. So even though it may seem business as usual in healthcare in the richer world, the system as a whole faces a number of serious challenges that fundamentally threaten its operation.

Table 1.1 Domains of actions to avoid serious adverse changes to the planet. (Reprinted by permission from Macmillan Publishers Ltd: Rockstrom J., Steffen W., Noone K., Persson A., Chapin F.S., Lambin E.F., et al. A safe operating space for humanity. Nature. 2009;461(7263):472–5. Copyright © 2009).

Planetary Boundaries

Earth system process	Parameters	Proposed boundary	Current value	Pre-industrial value
Climate change	Atmospheric carbon dioxide concentration (parts per million by volume)	350	387	280
Rate of biodiversity loss	Extinction rate (number of species per million species a year)	10	>100	0.1–1
Nitrogen cycle	Amount of N_2 removed from the atmosphere for human use (millions of tons per year)	35	121	0
Phosphorus cycle	Quantity of P flowing into oceans (millions of tons per year)	11	8.5–9.5	–1
Stratospheric ozone depletion	Concentration of ozone (Dobson unit)	276	283	290
Ocean acidification	Global mean saturation of aragonite in surface sea water	2.75	2.90	3.44
Global freshwater use	Consumption of freshwater by humans (km^3 per year)	4000	2600	415
Change in land use	Percentage of global land cover converted into cropland	15	11.7	Low
Atmospheric aerosol loading	Overall particulate concentration in the atmosphere on a regional basis		To be determined	
Chemical pollution	For example, amount emitted to or concentrations of persistent organic pollutants, plastics, endocrine disrupters, heavy metals and nuclear waste in the global environment, or the effects on ecosystem and functioning of Earth system thereof.		To be determined	

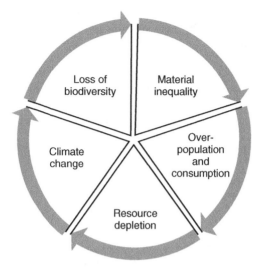

Figure 1.1 Five contemporary predicaments.

Five contemporary predicaments

In this section we take a wider look at the general human situation through the lens of five contemporary predicaments. These are predicaments we are unlikely to sort out with the same style of thinking that helped to create them, but which are explicable and potentially solvable from a sustainability perspective (Figure 1.1).

Material inequality

Although the diversity of the human situation means that inequalities in material wealth are inevitable, the *degree* of inequality within humanity is anomalous. More than a billion people currently live in what the World Bank defines as *extreme* poverty with an income of less than US$ 1.25 (£0.79) per day. Nearly half of the world's population lives on less than US$ 2 (£1.30) per day [6]. These income levels are not sufficient to meet basic human needs and are not remotely enough to support any advanced medical interventions in settings where people have to pay for services. For instance, a child developing insulin-dependent diabetes in an impoverished rural area may not receive insulin therapy because the cost would be beyond the means of the child's family (Case study 1.1).

In contrast, the world's wealthy are getting wealthier (as admittedly are the world's poor). The *United Nations University's* survey of the *World*

Case study 1.1   The fate of a child with diabetes in rural India

An eight-year-old girl called Sudha was admitted with DKA (diabetic ketoacidosis) soon after her diagnosis with Type 1 diabetes. On discharge, I explained to her parents the importance of insulin for survival. Sudha's poor and illiterate parents were very attentive. Finally her father asked:

'Doctor, if I understand you correctly, does Sudha have to take insulin injections every day for rest of life?'
'Yes.'
'What would happen if she stopped taking insulin?'
'Well, she would slip into coma and if left unattended, would die.'

Three months later Sudha had died. Her father had quite intentionally stopped giving her insulin. To the outsider he appears inhuman, cruel and criminal. But for him, the choice was between the starvation of his other children *versus* treatment of a diabetic child.

The average annual family income in India is Rs 50 000(£750/US$ 1185). The cost per annum for insulin and syringes alone is Rs 15 000 (£200/US$ 316). If blood glucose monitoring is included the cost is doubled.

With no health insurance cover, poor families find it difficult to commit over a quarter of their monthly income to the treatment of a diabetic child. The logic of poverty overpowers the logic of life.

Quoted, with permission, from a letter to one of the authors from Dr Sharad Pendsey, Consultant Diabetologist, Director, Diabetes Clinic and Research Centre, Nagpur, India and Managing Trustee, Dream Trust (www.dreamtrust.org).

Distribution of Household Wealth documents the divide with stark statistics [7]. In 2000, the richest 1% of the world adult population owned 40% of global assets, while the poorest half owned only 1%. Income correlates with success in all of the *United Nations' Millennium Development Goals*, including child health, universal education and putting an end to hunger [8]. The reasons for these differences in material wealth are complex and go far beyond the scope of this book. But although differences are material, the solutions may not be. This degree of material inequality indicates a profoundly dysfunctional global system. The United Nations, for instance, estimated in 1998 that the millennium goal of basic education for all could be attained by an additional global investment of US$ 6 billion (£3.8 billion).

In that same year people living in the USA spent US\$ 8 billion (£5 billion) on cosmetics, the people of Europe US\$ 11 billion (£6.9 billion) on ice cream and the world community US\$ 780 billion (£492 billion) on the military [9].

Population and consumption

In October 2011, the world population reached seven billion from a pre-industrial baseline of one billion, and the US Census Bureau estimates that the population will rise to nine billion by 2040 [10]. This growth equates to creating a new city of a million people every five days from now to 2050 [11]. One reason for this growth has been the *Green Revolution* (Chapter 6), which has been fuelled by new, energy-intensive ways of making nitrogenous fertilisers and the development of new disease and drought-resistant strains of grain [12]. An estimated 50% of people today depend for their calories on food grown using such artificial fertilisers. More people require more food, space, water and energy. Because some people consume much more than others, there is a good argument that the chief metric should be not population numbers *per se* but the *per capita* impact of each person on the earth's resources. The richest billion people on the planet consume, on average, 32 times as much as the remaining six billion [13]. The signs are that people in poorer countries now aspire to the sorts of lifestyles adopted in richer countries. Hence, any global transition to the western lifestyle will have a much greater impact than would be implied by population growth alone. Take, for example, an increasing appetite for meat in China and India (Chapter 6 gives an exposition of the environmental impact of animal protein). Rising consumption is, therefore, a greater threat than rising population. Fuelling such consumption is the rising tide of economic migration from poorer to richer economies, a tide that will certainly run stronger as climate change has its differential effects on the poorer world. This predicament lies in uneasy paradox with our first problem of inequality. We need the rich to consume less and the earth's poorer citizens to draw more on resources than they do already (these twin concepts of *contraction* and *convergence* are explored further in Chapter 3). An advantage of convergence is that family size tends to reduce as communities emerge from the extremes of poverty, easing population pressures [14].

Resource depletion

The resources of the earth, such as fossil fuels, are limited and even the energy we can extract each year from the sun is finite. In 2005, analysts reported that we had consumed half of all the earth's extractable reserves of conventional oil and gas [15]. They warned that remaining reserves would be more costly and more risky to exploit, as we saw for instance with the Deepwater Horizon disaster of 2010, in which an explosion led to oil gushing unchecked from the seabed and the biggest spill in United States' history [16]. This *peak oil* narrative holds true for conventional oils and gases, though the picture has become complicated because of the recent emergence of alternative hydrocarbon sources and extraction methods, such as shale oil and hydraulic fracturing. At current levels of consumption, supplies of conventional fuels are likely to be depleted by the end of the century, with much uncertainty over how alternative fuels, nuclear power and renewables will fill this energy void [15]. Experts predict substantive changes in the world economy as a result, including in the health sector [17]. If the supply of fossil fuels diminishes and prices rise, this will have severe implications for the delivery of healthcare, yet there is scant evidence that we are prepared for this transition. Imagine, for instance, running hospitals using 50% less energy than at present. Although such a situation might be desirable from a sustainability perspective, it would herald some fundamental changes in the way we realise our hospitals – changes that we need to start planning for now. The picture is set to be clarified in the next decade as the potential of alternative sources of hydrocarbons is established, though these will only worsen the problem of carbon emissions.

Water scarcity may turn out to be a bigger threat to global security than diminishing fossil fuels. Rivers such as the Rio Grande, the Nile, the Indus and China's Yellow River struggle to reach the sea throughout the year. We are taking water from rivers, lakes and aquifers faster than it can be replaced by the hydrological cycle [18]. Hydraulic 'fracking' for shale oil, our best hope for obtaining fossil fuels as conventional oil supplies decline, is an intensely thirsty process, pumping millions of gallons of water deep underground. Since fracking also forces chemicals underground, it has the potential not only to deplete but also contaminate supplies. The *UN Food and Agriculture Organisation (FAO)* estimates that 1.8 billion people will experience water scarcity by 2025. City communities such as La Paz in Bolivia, which draw their summer supplies from glacial melt water, are particularly vulnerable as glaciers recede due to global warming. Other resources in danger of depletion include rare earth metals such as neodymium (which makes the powerful magnets used in wind turbines), phosphates used in fertiliser production and uranium for nuclear fission. Like the Easter Islanders we are set to run short of the raw materials that underpin the processes of our civilisation.

Climate change

In October 2011, an independent and previously sceptical team of clima-tologists from Berkeley, California, confirmed findings from other centres that the average surface temperature of the earth has risen by one degree since 1950s [19]. This observation persists after adjusting for the possible confounding effects of *urban heat islands*, which are metropolitan areas that are considerably warmer than their surrounding rural areas. We know that the cause of this warming is mainly carbon dioxide from the burning of fossil fuels and that no other mechanism could account for the rapidity of the change (Chapter 2). The earth's poles are particularly sensitive. According to data from the *US National Centre for Atmospheric Research*, the extent of arctic sea ice has declined by 30% since 1979 [20]. With the melting of continental ice in Antarctica and Greenland comes the possibility of rising sea levels and the inundation of coastal communities. If evidence of current global warming is incontrovertible, it is much less certain how global warming will proceed as the century unfolds. We also do not know whether change will remain gradual or hit a tipping point as the earth system flips into a new and hotter state. The potential impacts of climate change on human health are huge and mediated particularly by loss of food security, through flood and drought, direct effects of extreme weather, expanding habitat for disease vectors such as malaria and the inevitable health consequences of mass migration from stricken areas [1]. Because of these pressing effects on health the whole of Chapter 2 is devoted to understanding the science of climate change and its impacts.

Loss of biodiversity

Perhaps we can rescue the climate, but once a species is extinct there is no going back. The current rate of extinction is thought to be between 100 and 1000 times the estimated background extinction rate (there are difficulties knowing for certain of the extinction of creatures such as ants at large in the Amazon basin). Many organisms are already 'functionally extinct' because they exist in numbers too small to have noticeable presence within their local ecosystems. Iconic examples include the Yangtze River Dolphin and the Iberian Lynx. The sociobiologist E.O. Wilson estimated in 2002 that, at current rates, one-half of all species on earth would be extinct in 100 years [21]. People seem remarkably unaware of the scale of what is happening – the greatest extinction event since the one 65 million years ago, when the dinosaurs and half of life on earth were wiped out by a meteorite or volcanic upheaval, or both. In our times a quarter of mammals, a third of those vulnerable amphibians, a quarter of corals and a quarter of freshwater fish are threatened [22]. Humanity has a long history of causing extinction of large mammals through direct predation; this still accounts for why so many species of fish and other cetaceans (marine mammals) are endangered. On land the mechanism of contemporary extinction has more to do with the depletion of habitats, as marshes are drained and forests cleared. Around half of the original six million square miles of tropical forest present in 1947 has now been destroyed. Current projections suggest that by 2030 we will be left with just 10% of the original coverage [23]. In specific pockets, such as Haiti, the tropical canopy is almost completely gone.

The impacts of such losses are incalculable and it takes particular imagination to grasp the impact of all this on human health. There is, for instance, the loss of plants and animals which might have turned out to have been of direct medicinal use. In his book *The Future of Life*, E.O. Wilson relates an anecdote in which a Bornean tree is discovered to yield a medicine active against HIV [21]. On returning to the remote swamp from where they gathered their sample, collectors found the tree had been felled and no more could be found. Luckily a specimen showed up in the Singapore Botanic Garden. What is harder to appreciate is how by removing species we 'damage ecosystems, collapse food webs and ultimately undermine the planetary life-support system on which our species depends' [24]. This is why we study systems in more depth in Chapter 3.

Crises in healthcare

So far we have defined five predicaments that confront us: inequalities, over-population with rising consumption, resource depletion, climate change and loss of biodiversity. We could add more, such as soil erosion, oceanic acidification and armed conflict. These predicaments are, of course, intimately interwoven. For example, fossil fuels have fuelled the development that stimulates population growth, which impacts on land use and, hence, biodiversity. We cannot solve these predicaments by simply doing more of what we are doing already. The threat to our lifestyle is our lifestyle. For instance, we will not be able to address the issues of material inequality by striving to bring the consumption levels of everyone up to the level of those in the wealthiest countries, as we are already exceeding the carrying capacity of the planet. These big picture predicaments are often removed from the daily work of healthcare professionals in the world's richer countries, though certainly not for those working in poorer ones.

Healthcare is a part of the global system like any other 'industry' and faces its own related suite of pressing predicaments [25]. Here we cite five *crises* in health, drawing on the *Oxford English Dictionary* definition of crisis as a 'time of difficulty, insecurity, and suspense' (Figure 1.2). Having defined these crises we go on to show, in this chapter and in the book as a whole, how sustainable healthcare offers at least the hope of solutions to the troubles of our times – solutions that the healthcare community will have a central role in bringing to life.

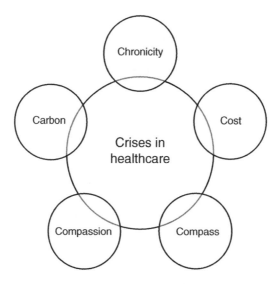

Figure 1.2 Crises in healthcare.

Crisis of chronicity

We know that the global population is growing. It is also aging. Japan, for instance, is estimated to be the 'oldest' nation that has ever existed, with one in ten of its citizens being over 75 years of age [13]. This demographic explains, in part, the shift in healthcare's orientation from the treatment of acute illness to the management of chronic disease. Chronic disease has always been with us but is emerging as the primary preoccupation of many healthcare systems, especially in higher-income countries. Take diabetes as a sentinel diagnosis, the prevalence of which is rising rapidly across the world. The number of people diagnosed with Type 2 diabetes in the United States rose by 33% between 1990 and 1998 [26]. Projections suggest that 29 million people will live with this condition in the United States by 2050 [27]. Diabetes is significant because it underpins trends in many other chronic health problems, such as heart disease and stroke. But why is diabetes becoming such a big a problem? The answer lies in a complex mix of demography, keener diagnosis and the worldwide emergence of another global health crisis – obesity. According to the World Health Organization (WHO), more people die from being overweight than from malnutrition [28]. The 500 million world citizens who are obese are at greater risk of diabetes, cancer, heart disease and a prodigious number of other ailments [29]. A particularly worrying trend is the emergence of obesity in children (Chapter 6). Healthcare systems across the world also face high burdens of cancer, autoimmune disease, respiratory disease and chronic infectious diseases such as HIV/AIDS and tuberculosis. Though we do not understand all the causes of these diseases, science has shown strong associations with modern sedentary lifestyles and the western diet. Being still is dangerous for our health. Never have we moved our bodies around the world so much without actually *moving* our bodies. In later chapters we will see how lifestyles and diet also contribute to our global environmental ills.

Crisis of cost

Richer nations invest vast and increasing sums of money in healthcare, most of it in the treatment of the chronic conditions referred to earlier. This expenditure continues at a time when most governments are seeking ways of spending and borrowing less. These two trends seem impossible to reconcile. European nations spend around 9% of their Gross Domestic Product (GDP) on healthcare; the United States spends an exceptional 17.4% [30]. The *US Congressional Budget Office* estimates that if the United States health budget continues to grow at current rates, the nation will be spending an unthinkable 31% of its GDP on healthcare by 2035 [31]. The high cost of healthcare is down to another complex mixture of factors as people live longer and accrue diagnoses. In the United States, for instance, one in two adults live with a chronic condition [32]. As medical science progresses, we find more things to do at higher cost. For instance, MRI scanning is now almost a routine procedure. And new drugs, especially for life-threatening disease, are often inordinately expensive: for example, 21 tablets (5 mg) of the myeloma treatment lenalidomide (*Revlimid*®), the subject of Adam Wishart's mordant documentary *The Price of Life* [33], cost the United Kingdom taxpayer an improbable £3570 (US$ 5643) [34]. In systems that are based on reimbursing physicians through private insurance companies, there are strong reverse incentives to cost containment. The more things health professionals do, the more they get paid. And the more insurance companies pay out to providers, the more they pass on in premiums. Predictably, these premiums can soon become unaffordable, so that in 2009 an estimated 50.7 million persons in the United States had no health insurance whatsoever [35]. In 2007, 625 of personal bankruptcies in the United States were due to medical fees that could not be paid [36].

Crisis of compass

If healthcare is unsustainably expensive in the rich world, we could at least hope that we are benefitting from the very latest scientific medicine and that this colossal expenditure is resulting in our better health. However, existing data do not uniformly support this optimistic hypothesis. On the contrary, evidence suggests that spending on healthcare is being invested in interventions that do not improve health. For instance, the *Dartmouth Atlas Project* has shown that patients who live in regions of the United States with a higher intensity pattern of care where they receive more visits, undergo more imaging examinations and are more frequently admitted to hospital, show no better survival rates than those living in regions with lower-intensity healthcare [37]. Billions are spend each year on coronary angioplasties and stents, yet a randomised controlled trial, published in April 2007 in the *New England Journal of Medicine*, found that these two procedures do not prolong life or prevent heart attacks in patients with stable coronary disease when compared to pharmaceutical approaches [38]. We also know from comparing data between nations that there is a poor correlation between expenditure on healthcare and longevity. For example, although Chileans and Americans enjoy similar average longevity (78.6 versus 78.3 years), healthcare spending per capita is, according to the Organisation for Economic Co-operation and Development (OECD), six times greater in the United States – and 25 times greater than in the famously low-cost Cuban system [39]. These data suggest that a high proportion of healthcare funds is being misspent, however well meaning and culturally reasonable the reasons behind this spending may be. This is, in part, due to the conflation of healthcare as part of a system of *care*, with healthcare as profit-driven *industry*. An independent review calculated that US pharmaceutical companies spent US$ 57.5 billion (£35.6 billion) in 2004 on promoting their products, giving them weighty influence over the delivery of care which is, inevitably, dominated by medication, even in less overtly commercialised systems [40]. And medication use is on the up in many clinical fields. For instance, the health service in England issued 39 million prescriptions for antidepressants in 2009, compared with 20.1 million in 1999, with no evidence that England is a happier country as a result [41].

Developments like these herald what we call the 'crisis of compass' – a crisis in the purpose and direction of the healthcare enterprise. And what if 'care' is not only ineffective but actually harmful [42]? In 2009, there were 1.2 million visits to US emergency rooms due to the misuse of prescribed medications [43]. Even when used correctly, medicines can cause grave harms which are often not initially apparent. According to research published in *The Lancet*, between 88 000 and 140 000 excess cases of serious coronary heart disease occurred in the United States over the market-life of the anti-inflammatory *rofecoxib (Vioxx®)* before it was withdrawn in 2004 [44]. Even health promotion may have unforeseen problems. For instance, the United Kingdom's £96 million per annum *National Breast Screening Programme* is mired in controversy as epidemiologists debate whether it causes more harm than good [45]. So judicious use of investigations, medications and surgery will remain at the heart of good medicine. But, as we argue in Chapter 10, just because some treatment is possible does not mean that it is desirable. The direction we advocate is toward better health with, paradoxically, *less healthcare*, putting a firmer emphasis on broad, holistic and mainly preventative interventions. A welcome and convenient truth is that such interventions, be they preventative or therapeutic, are also, typically, much kinder on the planetary system.

Crisis of compassion

One of the effects of delivering so much in healthcare is that health professionals have become very busy, with more patients having more 'done' during shorter hospital stays and clinic visits. Whilst our therapeutic systems have advanced, there has not been a corresponding advance in our ability to meet the human needs of those in our care. In fact, by some indicators, the clinical frontline of medicine is uncomfortably short of humanity. The UK's *Care Quality Commission* found in 2011 that almost half of hospitals did not meet basic standards for nutrition and dignity in the care of elderly patients (Box 1.1 shows some extreme examples) [46].

Of course, individual doctors and nurses would never condone these depressing stories of neglect, but neither can we argue that they are exceptional. In a medical culture that focuses primarily on targets, costs and demonstrable physical disease, the humanity of individual patient care can get marginalised. In United Kingdom hospitals, a culture of 'shift working' has risked the fragmentation of individual care, as has the demise of 'personal lists' in family medicine, where patients receive the majority of their care from a single doctor. When suffering from routine 'minor' medical problems, patients want easy access to care, but when they are more seriously sick there is no substitute for caring longitudinal relationships, physical touch and attention to basic things such as nutrition, pain relief, dignity and privacy. Empathic skills, such as the ability to convey a sense of hope, do not figure highly in the modern medical curriculum and the evidence, though conflicted, points to medical students becoming less empathic as they progress through the clinical years [47]. Health professionals in training are also not themselves always treated with dignity and compassion. According to correspondents to an *American Medical Association* article on humanism, hospital Residents reported sarcasm, dysfunctional mentors, excessively long working hours, ridicule when seeking time off due to ill health, and doctors driven by the need to pay off huge educational loans as being common problems [48]. It is a paradox that while compassion is a relatively unlimited and 'free' resource, we are busy driving it out of the system, draining our limited

Box 1.1   Quotations from 'We have been listening, have you been learning?' A report by the UK's Patients Association, 2011 [47].

'As you can imagine, my mother was horrified when she then turned up in hospital to discover dad sat beside his bed, quite literally sitting in his own faeces... In general during dad's time in hospital the nursing staff treated him as an object that they had to treat rather than a human being who should be included in his care and given the dignity that he deserves.'

'Even despite the often poor care he was receiving, my father had nothing but praise and gratitude for the people caring for him, and thanked them every time. However, to us he said that nobody cares in here what happens to you.'

'The horrible thing is that my mum was not alone in this situation. I witnessed the old lady in the bed opposite being left with a bowl of steaming hot soup which she pulled towards her before I could stop her, and poured it all over her upper legs. When the nurse was called she said she was busy and would be along in a minute! The lady suffered scalding to her legs and the doctor had to be called.'

'Mum has always been very particular about her appearance and personal hygiene. We found it hugely distressing to find her with dirty fingernails and dirty teeth. She also had food all over her clothes. We took an apron in with us for mum to wear when she ate, but it was barely used, unless a member of family was present.'

'She was not given a choice of food, calcichews for her bones, was not hoisted, not hydrated nor visited by a physiotherapist. Every day that I visited, the first thing she said was "Give me a drink!" It was only after I repeatedly insisted that my mother be offered these things that she gradually was given them over the weeks that followed.'

and 'expensive' resources in the process. We need to consider compassion as another element of quality in healthcare which may sit in healthy tension with indicators such productivity and throughput (Box 1.1).

Crisis of carbon

The carbon crisis is, understandably, not one recognised by most health professionals, but is in fact the crisis dealt with most directly in this book.

Healthcare consumes a great deal of energy on powering buildings, transport and the procurement of goods and services. The US Government's energy efficiency office, *Energy Star*, estimates that healthcare organisations in the United States consume US$ 8.8 billion (£5.5 billion) of energy per annum [49]. The *NHS Sustainable Development Unit (SDU)* attributes a full 3% of the carbon footprint in England to NHS-related activity [50]. While energy in Western societies appears to be plentiful and relatively cheap, we are facing two major challenges. Firstly, as stated earlier, the amount of energy at our disposal is likely to reduce as the century unfolds and the supply of cheap conventional fossil fuel begins to dwindle. Secondly, the effects of carbon dioxide emissions from fossil fuel consumption are powering climate change, and climate change is set to be a major challenge to global health (Chapter 2). So, healthcare is part of the problem in common with all other industries, and will also be called upon to be part of the solution. We come back to this predicament repeatedly in the book, particularly in Chapter 5 on 'low carbon care'.

And so we conclude this catalogue of crises: of chronicity, cost, compass, compassion and carbon. As with the global predicaments detailed above, these five crises in healthcare are, of course, strongly interconnected. While cheap energy has helped build the freedoms of modern culture, we have often built these without respect for the 'planetary boundaries' that constrain us. Our wit in harnessing fossil fuels has allowed the human population to grow and consume exponentially, but those same fuels have allowed our habits to become sedentary and our diets industrial. Healthcare has also become more industrialised, bringing affordable medicine to millions. But where unchecked, such healthcare has also led to grossly inflated costs and prolific activity that contributes directly to carbon emissions – often without confirmed benefits to human health.

As argued already, these predicaments cannot be solved by the system that created them. We need new ways of thinking and acting. The *sustainability paradigm* we offer here is of course not new; it has roots back to the conservationists of late nineteenth century America, such as John Muir and Henry David Thoreau. In the twenty-first century, sustainability has moved from the fringes to the mainstream of politics and academia. Many institutions now have cross-faculty institutes concerned wholly with responses to global environmental change [51]. Even the *British Medical Journal* carried 'The Greening of Medicine' as its cover headline in January 2012. Sustainability cannot be cast as a paradigm in the formal scientific sense. The predicaments it addresses are set on too broad a canvas and our response is as much about political will as scientific theory. What *is* new here is the application of these ideas at the heart of the modern medical enterprise, where up until recently they have been largely overlooked. And what *is* paradigmatic is that sustainability requires us to see all things differently, considering, for instance, not just *cost* but *carbon cost* of common things like medicines and clinic visits. We call this new way of seeing 'greening the medical gaze'.

Greening the medical gaze

In his influential book *The Birth of the Clinic* (1963), Michel Foucault (1926–1984) introduces the concept of the 'Medical Gaze', which refers to what doctors *see* when they view a patient and their predicament [52]. Seeing is more than a purely physiological process of light and neuronal pathways; it is a process of meaning-making. Health professionals learn how to 'read' visual objects such as microscope slides, X-rays, laboratory reports and even people for signs of diagnoses such as anaemia; we have borrowed this concept and applied it to our current situation, calling for an extension, or 'greening' of the medical gaze. While in the eighteenth century the medical gaze lighted upon the sick man in his home, in modern medicine it focuses on the results of clinical examination, blood tests and medical imaging in the clinic or hospital bed [53]. What we need now is a gaze that includes in its sweep how medicine sits within the Earth system as a whole, a subtle but revolutionary change of perspective from atomistic to holistic and from unbridled to sustainable development. This gaze does not supplant biomedicine. Rather it fits it into a necessarily bigger picture.

Sustainability defined

Environmental sustainability is too complex an idea to succumb to a unitary definition but, where the term is broached, consistent themes emerge. Sustainability is about looking after things now so that they can be enjoyed not only by us up to the end our lives but also by future generations. There is a sense of the long term, which is the antithesis of political expediency. The focus is on resilience, permanence and cycles rather than linear and unremitting growth: a steady-state approach rather than a frontier mentality. A seminal sustainability text is called, simply, *The Limits of Growth* [54]. Sustainability is concerned with relationships and how the different aspects of the earth system, such as climate, oceans, animals and plants, best work together. It is concerned, on one hand, with resources and how we can preserve them, and, on the other hand, with waste products and how we can best reduce or dispose of them. Thinking sustainably acknowledges planetary boundaries (Table 1.1) and seeks ways for humans to thrive within them. It views humans as guardians and stewards, not owners. The sustainability paradigm is values driven, seeing it as, for instance, unfair if the Earth's resources are exploited by some communities at the expense of others, including communities as yet unborn, with no choice or voice. We unpack the sustainability paradigm in more depth in Chapter 3, where we draw on the insights of *systems theory*. Sustainability then is not a single theory but a collection of tools, or lenses (theoretical, scientific, ethical and political), that bring possibilities into our field of vision that have until now gone unnoticed in our peripheral gaze – the perfect antidote to a 'crisis of compass'.

Up to now the medical sector has taken the gifts of the planetary system for granted. But by considering the sustainability perspective, health services will, for example, consider fossil fuel a precious resource that could provide hydrocarbons for medical plastics and pharmaceuticals into the deep future. To use fossil fuels as *fuels* does not make a lot of sense. If instead we go for active travel, walking and cycling instead of flying and driving we help keep oil and coal in its ideal environment – under the ground. And, at the same time, we improve our mood, become physically stronger and healthier, and stop emitting the exhaust gases which contribute to climate change and bad air in our cities. Observe how a single sustainability approach (active travel) is able to tackle a number of major predicaments at the same time. This is referred to as a *virtuous cycle*: what is good for the environment is also good for health (Chapter 3).

Social sustainability

This book focuses mainly on the environmental aspects of sustainability but UNESCO's campaign to promote sustainable development concentrates as much on the social as on the cultural. While financial and environmental sustainability are fairly intuitive concepts, social sustainability is more complex. It is about fostering communities that build capacity, develop skills, create social cohesion, improve health equity and champion resilience whilst at the same time looking after the physical environment. *The Young Foundation* stable of ventures, such as the UK's *Open University*, *Which? Magazine* and *NHS Direct*, is an excellent source of ideas and innovations in this area, accessible through its comprehensive website [55].

In Chapter 3 we explore the importance of diversity in the creation of resilient systems. Cultural diversity, like biodiversity, is something intrinsically worthy, which also contributes to the health of the whole. For instance, there are traditional approaches in medicine, such as Ayurveda, with its focus on diet, yoga and meditation, which might serve as models for the design of modern sustainable practice [56]. Like plants and animals, our languages are under threat of extinction, and with them cultural perspectives, developed over thousands of years, can die too. It is estimated that by 2050, half the world's 6000 languages will no longer have living speakers [57].

Social sustainability, then, is about preserving humanity's cultural heritage whilst encouraging social practices that enhance resilience, such as social justice, gender equality, religious tolerance, inter-generational equity, fair sharing of natural resources and basic education for all (in particular of women). The resulting social resilience has major medical implications, as research shows that people with strong social networks live longer healthier lives compared to those who are poorly connected in social terms [58]. Building communities is for this reason a legitimate part of the medical enterprise.

Sustainability and health services

Why should busy clinicians and managers devote time and energy to this agenda? Perhaps they are already convinced by the scientific evidence, or aware of the possibility of virtuous cycles and the need for energy resilience [50]. In the UK NHS there is also a statutory requirement for larger organisations to come in line with binding Government targets for an ambitious 80% reduction in carbon emissions by 2050 [59]. The *triple bottom line* is a succinct way of summarising the value of sustainability for the health professions. Firstly, sustainability can save money. Heat that is escaping from a poorly insulated building has to be paid for by someone. Avoiding unnecessary investigations means there is more money around to fund other more useful activities. Secondly, a sustainable approach leads to better health outcomes. If we focus on areas for improvement, such as better school meals, less advertising of processed food and health education for mothers, we might hold back the rising tide of obesity in children, who we know go on to become less healthy adults. Thirdly, sustainability nurtures the earth system. For instance, low carbon healthcare helps stem global warming and its attendant ills like drought and flooding. Remarkably, in 2010, the UK's Royal College of Physicians named sustainability as one of its seven domains of *quality* in healthcare [60]. The more we have explored sustainability the more clear it becomes that sustainable care is high quality care: lean, responsive and compassionate.

Ethics and exemplars

It would be wrong to caste sustainability as something managerial. The greening of the gaze is also about doing the *right* thing, an ethical position that brings out new aspects of old principles. For instance in the *Hippocratic Canon*, which forms the foundation of western medical ethics, we have the twin injunctions to do good and not to do harm. Sustainable healthcare applies these same ethics, not just to individual patients but to all life and the systems that sustain life. This is not lame environmental altruism, because we depend wholly on these systems for our survival. Whatever we do to the environment, we do ultimately to ourselves. Similarly, social justice takes on an ecological dimension. We need to ask ourselves: who owns the resources of the earth, how are they distributed and to what extent do we allow individuals to create wastes, such as carbon dioxide, that effect the whole of humanity?

Doctors have been instrumental in confronting many risks to health, for instance in their continuing tussle with the tobacco industry [61]. In an era of increasing mistrust in authority, nine in ten adults in the United Kingdom say they trust doctors to tell the truth [62]. This makes medics the most trusted profession in the United Kingdom, which brings with it not only important responsibilities to use this trust wisely but also significant leverage with individuals and in public debate. Although the number of health professionals embracing the implications of sustainability may still be relatively small, their impact based on this trust and leverage is growing steadily. Encouragingly, paradigmatic change is typically driven by the values and vision of individuals and small groups doing the groundwork, and waiting for a critical mass to emerge. Think of Semmelweis, derided for suggesting, in 1847, that puerperal fever in Vienna maternity hospitals was caused by contagion transmitted on the hands of medical students, in an era before the wide acceptance of Germ Theory. For those who are predisposed to think sustainably, engaging in these issues becomes not just an interest but a way of putting core values into practice.

Sustainability positive

Talk of boundaries, depletion, crisis and predicament underpins this opening chapter. Addressing these issues is the first and necessary step in a healing journey, an acceptance that all is not well. That process can be unwelcome and punctuated with denial and even resentment, as is discussed in Chapter 3. The word sustainability rightly conveys a sense of conservatism, preserving resources and reducing waste. But sustainability also unleashes huge opportunities for creative thought and healthcare entrepreneurship. We are drawn, for instance, to a model from rural China where health workers are paid when their patients are well but not when they are sick. Such new thinking will draw on resources whose supply is not likely to 'peak', resources such as knowledge, community, compassion and cooperation. A sustainable society will have less of some material things but more of other things, like civic trust, common purpose and individual and community wellbeing [63]. In short, we feel positive about the journey towards a sustainable future, even if the road ahead looks tortuous and uncertain.

About this book

In this chapter we have presented the idea of the sustainability paradigm as a necessary and quietly revolutionary response to the challenges of our time. We looked at predicaments in society as a whole and specifically in medicine, where we focused on the alliterative crises of chronicity, cost, compass, compassion and carbon. We have also given an outline of what sustainability means and boldly claim that it can deliver on the triple bottom line of quality of care, environmental protection and cost containment. The remainder of this book is about clothing these ideas in clear thinking, scientific evidence and practical ideas for transformative action. In Chapter 2 we take a non-technical look at climate science and review the current evidence for global warming and its likely impacts on health. In Chapter 3 we grapple with the concept of sustainability, drawing on systems thinking to arrive at a more nuanced definition, at the centre of which lies the idea of resilience. We also explore the difficulties of engaging with issues that are, on one hand, very unsettling and, on the other hand, seemingly remote. This chapter also introduces some of the necessary terminology of sustainable healthcare. The core ideas of the book culminate in Chapter 4 where we offer a vision for a sustainable health system. Chapters 5 to 11 are concerned with the practical application of these ideas to the organisation of clinical care, including chapters on food, transport, buildings and end-of-life care. We conclude, in Chapter 12, with a look at how health professionals can further their engagement with sustainability.

References

1. Costello, A., Abbas, M., Allen, A. *et al.* (2009) Managing the health effects of climate change: Lancet and University College London Institute for Global Health Commission. *Lancet*, **373** (9676), 1693–1733.
2. Diamond, J. (2006) *Collapse: How Societies Choose to Fail or Survive*. Penguin Books.
3. Armstrong, F. (2009) The Age of Stupid [DVD]. Dogwoof, London.
4. Rockstrom, J., Steffen, W., Noone, K. *et al.* (2009) A safe operating space for humanity. *Nature*, **461** (7263), 472–475.
5. CO_2 Now (Home) [Internet]. http://co2now.org/ [accessed 21 October 2011].
6. Measuring poverty – Wikipedia [Internet]. http://en.wikipedia.org/wiki /Measuring_poverty [accessed 13 October 2011].

7. UNU-WIDER (2008): World Distribution of Household Wealth [Internet]. http://www.wider.unu.edu/publications/working-papers/discussion-papers/2008/en_GB/dp2008-03/ [accessed 13 October 2011].

8. Dodd, R. and Cassels, A. (2006) Health, development and the Millennium Development Goals. *Annals of Tropical Medicine and Parasitology*, **100** (5–6):379–387.

9. UN Development Programme (1998) Human Development Report: Consumption and Human Development. UN Human Development Report Office (HDRO), New York.

10. US Census Bureau – International Programs: World Population [Internet]. http://www.census.gov/population/international/data/worldpop/table_population.php [accessed 26 January 2012].

11. The Royal Society (2012) People and the planet [Internet]. http://royalsociety.org/policy/projects/people-planet/ [accessed 29 May 2012].

12. Smil, V. (2004) *Enriching the Earth: Fritz Haber, Carl Bosch, and the Transformation of World Food Production*. MIT Press, MA.

13. Pearce, F. (2010) *Peoplequake: Mass Migration, Ageing Nations and the Coming Population Crash*. Eden Project Books, UK.

14. Myrskyla, M., Kohler, H-P. and Billari, F.C. (2009) Advances in development reverse fertility declines. *Nature*, **460** (7256):741–743.

15. Heinberg, R. (2005) *Party's Over: Oil, War and the Fate of Industrial Societies*, 2nd edn. Clairview Books, Forest Row, UK.

16. Campbell, T.C. (2005) Understanding Peak Oil. *Permaculture Magazine*, **46**, 3–6.

17. Raffle, A.E. (2010) Oil, health, and health care. *British Medical Journal*, **41**, c4596–c4596.

18. Pearce, F. (2007) *When The Rivers Run Dry: What Happens When Our Water Runs Out?* Eden Project Books, UK.

19. Berkeley Earth Surface Temperature (© 2011) [Internet]. http://berkeleyearth.org/ [accessed 21 October 2011].

20. Kay, J.E., Holland, M.M. and Jahn, A. (2011) Inter-annual to multi-decadal Arctic sea ice extent trends in a warming world. *Geophysical Research Letters*, 38 [Internet]. http://nsidc.org/icelights/2011/08/24/climate-change-or-variability-what-rules-arctic-sea-ice/ [accessed 21 October 2011].

21. Wilson, E.O. (2003) *The Future of Life*. Abacus, UK.

22. International Union for Conservation of Nature and Natural Resources – The IUCN Red List of Threatened Species [Internet]. http://www.iucnredlist.org/ [accessed 21 October 2011].

23. Mongillo, J. (2000) *Encyclopedia of environmental science*. Oryx Press, Phoenix, AZ.

24. Lynas, M. (2011) *The God Species: How the Planet Can Survive the Age of Humans*. Fourth Estate, London.

25. Peters, D. (2005) Bio-medicine in crisis: cost, cure, compassion and commitment. *Journal of Holistic Healthcare*, **2**, 2.

26. Mokdad, A.H., Ford, E.S., Bowman, B.A. *et al.* (2000) Diabetes trends in the U.S.: 1990–1998. *Diabetes Care*, **23** (9), 1278–1283.

27. Boyle, J.P., Honeycutt, A.A., Narayan, K.M.V. *et al.* (2001) Projection of Diabetes Burden Through 2050. *Diabetes Care*, **24** (11), 1936–1940.

28. Obesity and overweight [Internet]. World Health Organization. http://www
    .who.int/mediacentre/factsheets/fs311/en/index.html [accessed 27 October
    2011].
29. Reilly, J.J., Methven, E., McDowell, Z.C. *et al.* (2003) Health consequences of
    obesity. *Archives of Disease in Childhood*, **88** (9), 748–752.
30. OECD – Health at a Glance 2011: OECD indicators [Internet]. http://www
    .oecd-ilibrary.org/sites/health_glance-2011-en/index.html?contentType=/ns
    /Book,/ns/StatisticalPublication&itemId=/content/book/health_glance-2011-en
    &containerItemId=/content/serial/19991312&accessItemIds=&mimeType=text
    /html [accessed 26 January 2012].
31. Congressional Budget Office (2007) The Long-Term Outlook of Health Care
    Spending. Congressional Budget Office, Washington, DC.
32. Centers for Disease Control and Prevention (CDC) – Chronic Diseases and
    Health Promotion [Internet]. http://www.cdc.gov/chronicdisease/overview
    /index.htm#ref2 [accessed 27 October 2011].
33. *New Scientist* (2009) Opinion– The Price of Life: When healthcare meets
    money [Internet]. http://www.newscientist.com/article/dn17323-the-price-of-
    life-when-healthcare-meets-money.html [accessed 27 October 2011].
34. *British National Formulary* (2011) Gardners Books, Eastbourne, UK.
35. US Assistant Secretary for Planning and Evaluation (ASPE) (2007)
    Overview of the Uninsured in the US: Analysis of the 2007 CPS [Internet].
    http://aspe.hhs.gov/health/reports/07/uninsured/index.htm [accessed 17 March
    2012].
36. Himmelstein, D.U., Thorne, D., Warren, E. and Woolhandler, S. (2009) Medical
    bankruptcy in the United States, 2007: results of a national study. *American
    Journal of Medicine*, **122** (8), 741–746.
37. Wennberg, J.E. (2010) *Tracking Medicine: A Researcher's Quest to Understand
    Health Care*. OUP USA.
38. Boden, W.E., O'Rourke, R.A., Teo, K.K. *et al.* (2007) Optimal Medical Therapy
    with or without PCI for Stable Coronary Disease. *New England Journal of Medicine*,
    356, 1503–1516.
39. OECD – OECD Health Data 2011 – Frequently Requested Data [Internet].
    http://www.oecd.org/document/16/0,3746,en_2649_37407_2085200_1_1_1
    _37407,00.html [accessed 29 March 2012].
40. Gagnon, M-A. and Lexchin, J. (2008) The Cost of Pushing Pills: A New Estimate
    of Pharmaceutical Promotion Expenditures in the United States. *PLoS Medicine*,
    5 (1), e1.
41. NHS Business Services Authority (Home) [Internet]. http://www.nhsbsa.nhs.uk/
    [accessed 17 March 2012].
42. Kilo, C.M. and Larson, E.B. (2009) Exploring the harmful effects of health care.
    Journal of the American Medical Association, **302** (1), 89–91.
43. Goodnough, A. (2011) Prescription Drugs Abuse Sends More People to Hospi-
    tal. *The New York Times* [Internet]. http://www.nytimes.com/2011/01/06/health
    /06drugs.html?_r=2&ref=us [accessed 26 January 2012].
44. Graham, D.J., Campen, D., Hui, R. *et al.* (2005) Risk of acute myocardial
    infarction and sudden cardiac death in patients treated with cyclo-oxygenase

2 selective and non-selective non-steroidal anti-inflammatory drugs: nested case–control study. *Lancet*, **365** (9458), 475–481.

45. Autier, P., Boniol, M., Gavin, A. and Vatten, L.J. (2011) Breast cancer mortality in neighbouring European countries with different levels of screening but similar access to treatment: trend analysis of WHO mortality database. *British Medical Journal*, **343**, d4411–d4411.

46. Care Quality Commission (2011) The state of health care and adult social care in England: an overview of key themes in care in 2010/11. The Stationery Office, London.

47. Hojat, M., Mangione, S., Nasca, T.J. *et al.* (2004) An empirical study of decline in empathy in medical school. *Medical Education*, **38** (9), 934–941.

48. American medical Association – Has Medicine Lost Its Compassion And Humanism? [Internet]. http://www.ama-assn.org/ama/pub/education-careers/graduate-medical-education/question-of-month/medicine-lost-compassion.page? [accessed 30 October 2011].

49. ENERGY STAR – ENERGY STAR for Healthcare: [Internet]. http://www.energystar.gov/index.cfm?c=healthcare.bus_healthcare [accessed 2 February 2012].

50. NHS Sustainable Development Unit (2008) NHS England Carbon Emissions Carbon Footprinting Report. NHS Sustainable Development Unit, Cambridge, UK.

51. Hoare, A., Cornell, S., Bertram, C. *et al.* (20080 Teaching against the grain: multi-disciplinary teamwork effectively delivers a successful undergraduate unit in sustainable development. *Environmental Education Research*, **14** (4), 469–481.

52. Foucault, M. (2003) *The Birth of the Clinic: An Archaeology of Medical Perception*, 3rd edn. Routledge.

53. Jewson, N.D. (1976) The Disappearance of the Sick-Man from Medical Cosmology, 1770–1870. *Sociology*, **10**, 225–244.

54. Meadows, D.H., Randers, J. and Meadows, D.L. (2004) *The Limits to Growth: The 30-year Update*, revised ed. Earthscan Ltd, London.

55. The Young Foundation – A centre for Social Innovation [Internet]. http://www.youngfoundation.org/ [accessed 13 May 2012].

56. Singh, J., Desai, M.S., Pandav, C.S. and Desai, S.P. (2012) Contributions of ancient Indian physicians - Implications for modern times. *Journal of Postgraduate Medicine*, **58** (1), 73–78.

57. Harrison, K.D. (2008) *When Languages Die: The Extinction of the World's Languages and the Erosion of Human Knowledge*. OUP USA.

58. Putnam, R. (2001) *Bowling Alone: The Collapse and Revival of American Community*. Simon & Schuster Ltd.

59. Climate Change Act 2008 – Wikipedia [Internet]. http://en.wikipedia.org/wiki/Climate_change_act [accessed 4 November 2011].

60. Atkinson, S., Ingham, J., Cheshire, M. and Went, S. (2010) Defining quality and quality improvement. *Clinical Medicine*, **10** (6), 537–539.

61. Hymowitz, N. (2011) Smoking and cancer: a review of public health and clinical implications. *Journal of the National Medical Association*, **103** (8), 695–700.

62. Ipsos MORI (2011) Doctors are most trusted profession – politicians least trusted [Internet].   http://www.ipsos-mori.com/researchpublications/researcharchive /2818/Doctors-are-most-trusted-profession-politicians-least-trusted.aspx [accessed 4 November 2011].

63. Wilkinson, R. and Pickett, K. (2010) *The Spirit Level: Why Equality is Better for Everyone*. Penguin Books.

Chapter 2 **Climate science in context**

In this chapter

- Making sense of environmental science
- The impact of humans on the environment
- Effects of environmental change on health
- A call to action

Climate change may well be the biggest global health threat of the twenty-first century [1]. The scientific evidence suggests that the impacts of climate change are likely to be severe and that we almost certainly will not be able to avoid at least some of these. Only when we believe in the gravity of the situation and the benefits of action (both immediate and longer term) will we truly be able to engage with this important issue, support low-carbon policies and leave a heritage of which we can be proud. To quote David Attenborough: 'No one will protect what they do not first care about'.

In this chapter we look at the evidence behind the changing climate. Without wanting to infuse fear or guilt, we try to outline what we currently know for certain, while also pointing out those areas where uncertainties exist. We give a synopsis here and concentrate on the issues and facts that we need for a basic understanding of the science, referring to original sources as appropriate. We list key reports and sources for further information at the end of the chapter for those who want more detail.

Dealing with crises

Health professionals are well used to dealing with clinical crises. In the emergency room or in primary care settings, they sometimes have to make urgent clinical decisions without the benefit of a formal diagnosis. To give an example, an acutely feverish child presenting in UK primary care is likely to be suffering from a non-specific viral infection. Add a

Sustainable Healthcare, First Edition. Knut Schroeder, Trevor Thompson, Kathleen Frith and David Pencheon.
© 2013 John Wiley & Sons, Ltd. Published 2013 by John Wiley & Sons, Ltd.

non-blanching rash and a carer's report of fast deterioration over a few hours, and meningococcal disease – a medical emergency –enters the list of likely differential diagnoses. Rather than waiting for verification through a formal laboratory diagnosis which can take hours, judicious clinicians will administer antibiotics immediately to avoid serious illness or even death. Failing to spot and act on the typical symptoms and signs of meningococcal disease would rightly be considered negligent. Where there is no real consensus about what an action (or failure to act) may cause to the environment or the wider population, the *precautionary principle* can help with making such decisions by postulating that those taking the action – or avoiding it – must provide proof that they are *not* causing harm in doing so.

In the same way as high fever can be a 'red flag' for serious illness in a child, do terrestrial heat waves and temperature records indicate a situation in need of immediate and drastic action? The frequency and severity of such events are forcing us to consider the underlying problems that our world faces. For example, in 2011 a heat wave affected the Eastern United States and Canada, causing Newark, New Jersey, to record its highest ever temperature at 42°C (108°F), one of 220 records broken in the United States during this period. Does this mean the planet is 'ill'? Do any other 'symptoms and signs' support this notion? If so, can we do anything about it? And what might happen to us and the planet if we do not? We try to attempt answering these and other questions in the following sections. We have given greater weight to evidence that is based on rigorously and independently conducted research. Even panels of experts may not be entirely immune to conflicts of interest [2] but the assessments used for this book are the most rigorous available.

Making sense of environmental science

Environmental science brings together various disciplines, such as atmospheric science, biology, chemistry, ecology, geology, meteorology, physics and soil science. Being aware of the complexity of research in this area can help us appreciate the interpretative challenges that climate scientists face. Environmental science also uses various research methods. For example, some evidence in this field is based on long-term observations that help clarify the current situation. These data are also being used to create computer models that try to predict what may happen in the future. Consequently, there are limitations to the science of prediction and projection (we come back to these later in this chapter), as models often have to take into account a large number of as yet not fully understood variables. For instance, scientists remain uncertain as to whether cloud cover has a net cooling or warming effect. So to be credible, environmental science needs to state clearly what is happening now and what may or may not happen in the future – and distinguish very clearly between these two.

The impact of humans on the environment

Ecologist Eugene Stoermer and atmospheric chemist Paul Crutzen, motivated by the extent and growing evidence for the effect that human activities have on the Earth's ecosystems, coined a new informal geological term in the year 2000 and called this age of planetary change the *Anthropocene* (Chapter 1). Global climate change is widely regarded as the most urgent environmental issue in the *Anthropocene* because it affects humans around the globe, particularly with regard to food security and access to clean water [3–7].

What is the evidence for global climate change?

The earth's climate is constantly changing. The planet has had ice ages as well as longer warm periods, but there is increasing evidence that global temperatures are currently rising at unprecedented rates due to human activity. The research evidence for this warming has been compiled by the Intergovernmental Panel on Climate Change (IPCC), a team that involves over 1000 scientists from around the globe. In its 2007 *4th Assessment Report*, the IPCC concluded that 'warming of the climate system is unequivocal' [6]. Any remaining doubts about rising earth surface temperatures were dispelled in 2011 by the Berkeley Earth Surface Temperature Study, which has created a data set combining 1.6 billion temperature reports from 15 pre-existing data archives [8]. This study presents secure evidence of an average rise in world land temperatures of approximately 1°C since the mid-1950s.

Surface temperature is not the only marker of global warming. The UK Met Office compiled, in 2011, results for other climate indicators from over 20 international institutions. Using a variety of resources and independent analysts to confirm the findings, data clearly show a rise in global average temperature (Figure 2.1), increases in ocean water temperatures, rising sea levels, as well as shrinking of the arctic sea ice, glaciers and Northern hemisphere snow cover [9].

The link between temperature changes and carbon dioxide

Various factors influence climate. Changes in the Earth's orbit, volcanic eruptions, sunspot activity and atmospheric concentration of greenhouse

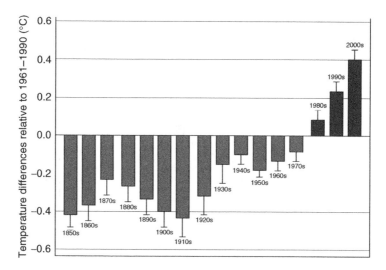

Figure 2.1 Observed global average temperature for each decade from 1850 to 2009 relative to 1961–1990 [9]. (Reproduced with permission from the UK Met Office. Contains public sector information licensed under the Open Government Licence v1.0.) [9]

gases (GHGs) all alter the earth's energy balance. But what we are seeing now is not such natural variation. Concentrations of carbon dioxide have risen by more than 35% since the beginning of industrialization and are now at the highest level for at least 800 000 years. And between 1970 and 2004, GHG levels increased by 70% [6]. The evidence leaves no doubt that the burning of fossil fuels, coupled with large-scale deforestation, has affected the composition of the Earth's atmosphere considerably. How do we know this?

C. David Keeling of the Scripps Institution of Oceanography started to measure the concentration of carbon dioxide at the Mauna Loa observatory on Hawaii in 1958 [10]. These data provide the longest continuous record of direct measurements of carbon dioxide in the atmosphere and clearly show a steady rise in carbon dioxide concentrations in recent decades (Figure 2.2). Radioisotope studies prove that this 'new' carbon dioxide is of fossil fuel origin. The graph's saw-tooth appearance is due to the seasonal uptake of carbon dioxide by plants in the northern hemisphere summer.

To learn about atmospheric carbon dioxide levels in the distant past, scientists drill deep down into the ice of the Antarctic and measure the composition of tiny bubbles of air trapped in these ice cores [11]. Evidence from studies like these shows that atmospheric carbon dioxide has been

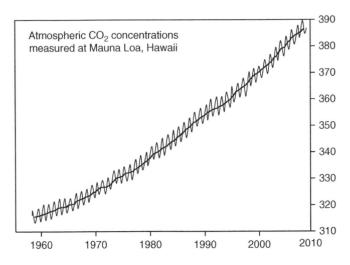

Figure 2.2 Monthly mean atmospheric carbon dioxide at Mauna Loa Observatory, Hawaii. (Reproduced with permission from Dr. Pieter Tans, NOAA/ESRL (www.esrl.noaa.gov/gmd/ccgg/trends/) and Dr. Ralph Keeling, Scripps Institution of Oceanography (scrippsco2.ucsd.edu/).) [10]

closely linked with Antarctic temperatures over a period of 800 000 years. Current levels of carbon dioxide are much higher than at any time over this period (Figure 2.3).

As in medicine, *association* does not prove *causation*. However, atmospheric carbon dioxide and global warming are linked by a well-demonstrated climatic mechanism known as the *greenhouse effect*.

The greenhouse effect

Clinicians learn how various gases and aerosols affect the human body, particularly during surgery or in intensive care. Similarly, to understand climate change, we need to know about the important role that gases play in the earth's climate.

When radiation from the sun at the higher frequencies of visible light enters the atmosphere and warms the Earth's surface, the resulting energy is emitted through infrared thermal radiation at lower frequencies. Greenhouse gases have the capability of absorbing this infrared radiation, returning some of this energy back to the lower atmosphere and the planet's surface (Figure 2.4). As a result, the earth maintains its temperature – similar to a greenhouse – by trapping infrared radiation and stopping it escape into space. Without this gaseous cloak and the Earth's atmosphere, which reflects ultraviolet light

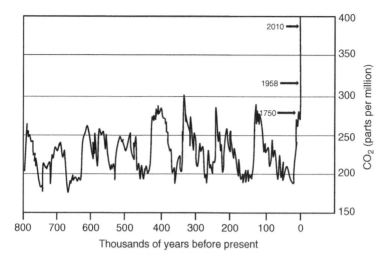

Figure 2.3   Atmospheric carbon dioxide levels – 800 000 years ago to present time. (Based on data from Luethi *et al.* [11].)

from the sun, temperatures would soar during the day before dropping well below freezing at night.

We know that carbon dioxide, which is a product of burning fossil fuels in homes, coal-fired power stations and combustion engines (e.g. in cars and aeroplanes), is an important greenhouse gas. Generation of electricity and heat was by far the main contributor to carbon dioxide emissions in 2009, leading to 41% of the world's carbon dioxide emissions [12]. But carbon dioxide is not the only GHG implicated in the greenhouse effect. Methane (CH_4), for example, has a much higher warming potential than carbon dioxide (by about a factor of 25) and is produced in agriculture, landfill sites and melting permafrost, though in much smaller quantities than carbon dioxide. Other gases, such as nitrous oxide (N_2O) or refrigerant gases, are even more potent (300 times for N_2O and even higher for the refrigerant gases), but are emitted in even smaller amounts. Because multiple greenhouse gases may be generated at the same time, it's their *combined impact* that counts. This is referred to as *carbon dioxide equivalent (CO_2e)*: the amount of carbon dioxide that would have the same effect.

Greenhouse gases contribute to maintain the planet's surface air temperatures around an average of 15°C (59°F), with peaks and troughs much less extreme than they would be without a gas-filled atmosphere. So, as the levels of these gases rise, so does the average temperature.

The naturally occurring feedback loops and homeostatic mechanisms that respond to variations in atmospheric carbon dioxide (such as buffering by sea

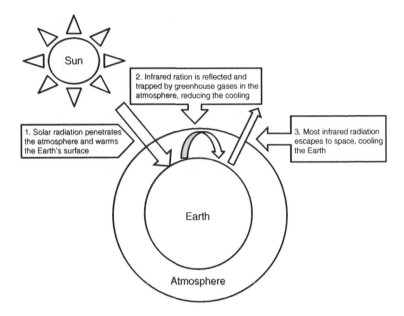

Figure 2.4 Effect of greenhouse gases.

water) are not powerful enough to cope with the rapid and large scale changes we are currently experiencing. As a result, carbon dioxide levels are rising and there is now overwhelming evidence for *global warming* from observations of increases in global average air and ocean temperatures, extensive melting of snow and ice, and a rise in global average sea levels when compared with past baseline measures obtained through samples from ice cores, tree rings or sediment [8, 13].

Human-generated climate change

As a result of human activities since around 1750, global atmospheric concentrations of carbon dioxide, methane and nitrous oxide have increased markedly and now are far higher than pre-industrial values, based on findings from ice cores covering a period of many thousands of years [13]. By September 2011, concentrations of carbon dioxide in the atmosphere have risen from pre-industrial levels of 250 to 389 ppm [14], and scientists almost unanimously believe that the rise in average global temperature cannot be explained unless they include such GHGs. Fossil fuel use and changes in land use are largely responsible for the global increases in carbon dioxide levels, whereas agriculture in particular has led to the rises in methane and nitrous oxide levels. This overwhelming evidence led the IPCC to conclude that 'most of the observed increase in global average temperatures since the mid-20th century is very likely due to the observed increase in anthropogenic carbon dioxide and other greenhouse gas concentrations' [13].

Greenhouse gases and associated pollutants not only affect the world's climate but also have a direct effect on people's health. A meta-analysis and analysis of a cohort study of just over 350 000 people in 66 US cities conducted by an international team of researchers showed that certain greenhouse pollutants, such as sulfate, black carbon and ozone, increased the risk of death [15]. The authors concluded that reducing black carbon and ozone precursors would lead to almost immediate health benefits.

Estimating climate change: modelling the future

If greenhouse gases continue to increase, climate models predict that mean global temperatures may rise between 2 and 5°C above 1990 levels by the end of this century [4, 6]. But considerable uncertainty still exists about how much temperatures will change, at what rate and what the exact effects will be. James Lovelock, the originator of *Gaia Theory*, argues that climate change is unlikely to be gradual as often depicted in IPCC projections, but rather that the earth will reach a 'tipping point' and flit into a much hotter state [16].

Worryingly, climate change itself may incur further warming through amplifying feedback mechanisms (Chapter 3). For example, a reduction in the area of ice sheets reduces the fraction of solar radiation reflected by the earth (also known as *albedo*, or *reflection coefficient*), so leading to further warming [17]. And melting of the arctic permafrost can release methane stored away in the soil [4, 6, 18]. Although soil and plants (algae, for example) have the capacity to absorb carbon dioxide to a certain level, they will be less likely to do so at higher temperatures. In addition, changes in the amount of water vapour or the consistency and distribution of clouds may reduce or amplify climate change [19]. The effects of climate change are far from clear because of uncertainties around the effects of feedback loops, 'tipping points' and non-linear change. In the worst case, this could lead to a catastrophic outcome, which has been called *runaway climate change* [4].

To simulate past climate and project changes in global climate in the future, scientists use mathematical models that take into account diverse parameters, such as atmospheric pressure, oceanic acidity or forest cover. *Projections* are distinguished from *predictions* in that they may also involve assumptions about human activities, such as agriculture, population dynamics and technological developments, which means that they are subject to substantial uncertainty [20]. Scientists have to make certain

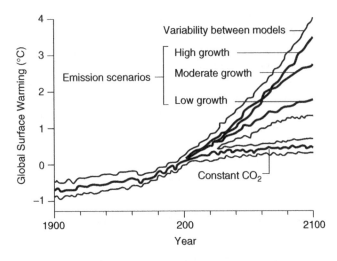

Figure 2.5 Increase in global surface warming using different emissions scenarios. (Modified, with permission, from [20] Intergovernmental Panel on Climate Change. Climate Change 2007: Synthesis Report. Contribution of Working Groups I, II and III to the Fourth Assessment Report of the Intergovernmental Panel on Climate Change, Figure SPM.5, right panel. IPCC, Geneva, Switzerland.)

assumptions, so any predictions can only be *estimates*, which is why predictions vary between institutions and the models being used.

Like medical research, the science of climate change has made enormous progress in the past two decades [19]. This is due to better and more effective use of long-term climate data, the increasing number of climate observations, more advanced measurement techniques, improved climate simulations and more powerful computing technology. All this has helped to strengthen the case for attributing climate change to human activity and reduce uncertainties.

Despite these uncertainties, there is high agreement and strong evidence that over the next few decades global GHG emissions will continue to increase by 25–90%, even with current climate change mitigation policies and levels of sustainable development [6]. Even if concentrations of GHGs and aerosols stayed constant at year 2000 levels, scientists would still expect further warming of around 0.1°C per decade. Figure 2.5 illustrates the variability of predicted global surface warming between models that use different emission scenarios.

In addition to temperature and atmospheric carbon dioxide levels, we can also observe changes in other climate variables. For example, scientists have observed a decline of about 2.4 million square kilometres of Arctic summer sea ice since the late 1970s; this is an area larger than Greenland [9]. Due to the time scales associated with climate processes and feedbacks, we are likely to see continued global warming and sea level rise for centuries, even if we manage to stabilise greenhouse gas concentrations and stop the emission of greenhouse gases immediately [6]. But as the predictions indicate, we have some choice over the matter. If the world moves to using more low-carbon and sustainable energy, the global temperature is expected to rise by 1.8°C (likely range 1.1–2.9°C) by the end of the century. Should we put less emphasis on sustainability, the likely rise is thought to be around 4.0°C (likely range 2.4–6.4°C), with abrupt or irreversible impacts on ecosystems becoming much more likely.

Climate change denial

Some people remain in denial about the effect that human activities have on the planet, believing that certain claims made by environmental scientists are exaggerated or false (Chapter 3 gives more on the psychology of climate change denial) [21]. They may hold the view that more evidence is needed before we should curb the activities of populations and economies, particularly where this leads to perceived inconvenience or costs. Some health professionals, perhaps those who are being overly sceptical by nature, may also hold such views.

This, perhaps, is not too surprising, because many people working in the health sector have learnt to be sceptical – and for good reason. New medical research emerges all the time, so clinicians, for example, must know whether they can trust the results of new studies and whether these are relevant for treating their patients. Modern medical schools teach students critical appraisal skills to help them decide whether new scientific evidence should lead to a change in practice or not. Being able to tell the difference between studies (or systematic reviews of studies) that should lead to a change in practice and those that do not is an important skill. Studies may be of poor quality, have biases, or have used study participants that are different from those that people see in their routine clinical practice, which are of course all issues that we need to consider when judging the quality and relevance of a study. In medicine, as in any other science, practice often only changes if there is an emerging 'body of evidence' that leads to a 'tipping point' in opinion, that is, a situation in which the perceived costs and disadvantages of not acting are greater than those connected with acting. A good example is tobacco control, which has parallels to the climate change debate: both deal with serious challenges, both are influenced by vested interests and 'junk science', and interventions in both areas have emerged only slowly despite ever growing evidence supporting the need for urgent action [22]. Though there still is an important difference: with smoking the costs are personal and local, whereas the consequences of climate change affect much larger populations.

We have certainly reached this 'tipping point' in the field of climate science, and in this chapter we have tried to demonstrate why this is the case. However, there may be forces working in the background trying to disrupt this consensus. For example, a review in 2008 of 141 environmentally sceptical books published between 1972 and 2005 shows that over 92% of these books were linked to conservative think tanks [23]. Interestingly, when the authors looked more closely, they found that 90% of these think tanks (which were largely funded by wealthy conservative foundations and corporations) supported environmental scepticism. This led the researchers to conclude that environmental scepticism may, in many cases, be fuelled by small powerful groups aiming to oppose environmentalism and weaken governmental efforts to protect the environment for their own gain.

Effects of climate change on ecosystems and health

We have by now established that climate change is indeed a reality. In this next section we explore the implications of these changes for the earth system and human health [3, 6, 19, 24].

The importance of a healthy environment for human health

From a human perspective, we depend on functioning ecosystems, because the natural environment supplies resources and processes that are essential to human health [24]. Such benefits, like clean drinking water or the decomposition of organic waste, are known as *ecosystem services*. Various types of ecosystems, such as forests, coastal and mountain regions, drylands and cultivated areas, can provide different combinations of 'services' to human populations. These ecosystems are now under threat from climate change [25]. The 2004 *Millennium Ecosystem Assessment*, a four-year study by the United Nations involving an international team of 1300 scientists, grouped ecosystem services into four groups [24]:

1. **Provisioning** – such as production of clean air, drinking water and food.
2. **Regulating** – such as controlling diseases and climate.
3. **Supporting** – such as pollination of crops and nutrient cycles.
4. **Cultural** – such as positive recreational and spiritual effects.

This study re-affirms how much we depend on the natural environment to provide us with the conditions for a healthy and secure life of decent quality – something that is easily forgotten in modern urban living. The report also points out that over the past 50 years humans have caused ecosystems to change rapidly and extensively to meet our growing needs for clean water, food, fuel, fibre and timber. As a result, the diversity of life on Earth is under serious threat and has in some respects already been lost (Chapter 1). Although changes in ecosystems (because of land cultivation) have helped to improve the lives of billions, they have a cost attached to them in the form of degrading ecosystems, climate change and increasing poverty for certain groups of people. For example, approximately one quarter (24%) of Earth's terrestrial surface has been cultivated, about 40% of coral reefs have been destroyed or badly degraded, an estimated 35% of mangroves have been lost and at least one quarter of marine stocks are over-harvested [25].

A report for the Countryside Recreation Network in 2005 provides evidence that nature can also provide more subtle, positive contributions to our health, such as recovering better from pre-existing stresses or problems, and helping us to concentrate and think more clearly [26]. The evidence is growing that we clearly and heavily depend on functioning ecosystems [27]. For this and many other reasons we must not take them for granted, even if they appear to be 'for free' [28].

Effects of climate change on health

The World Health Organization estimates that modifiable factors in air, water, soil and food already cause a quarter of the global disease burden, and over a third of the childhood burden [29]. For example, extreme weather events, malnutrition and changing patterns of infectious diseases in combination with migration and population growth will have (and to a certain extent already have) a great impact on human health globally. This is on the back of a pre-existing global health crisis, which sees millions of children die each year and 1.5 billion people not having access to clean drinking water. It is estimated that climate change has already caused the loss of around 5.5 million disability adjusted life years (DALY, a measure of overall disease burden which is expressed as the number of years lost due to ill-health, disability or early death) in the year 2000 alone [1].

People living in low-income countries may find it particularly difficult to adapt to changes in climate and their consequences, and these countries are likely to suffer the highest impact [6]. Even in higher-income countries, vulnerable people like those on low incomes, young children and older individuals will also be at increased risk, depending on the location of a country. Other important vulnerable groups of people include people living

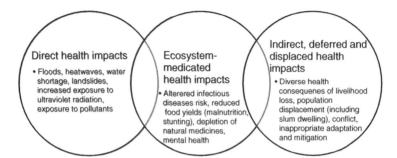

Figure 2.6 Effects of environmental changes on human health. (Data from McMichael *et al.* [30].)

in low-lying coastal areas and those with chronic illnesses. These are the populations and people who are least resilient, and climate change no doubt will exacerbate already existing inequalities.

The effects of environmental changes, such as climate change, and environmental damage (for example forest clearing, freshwater depletion or damage to ecosystems) on human health of populations are complex and interdependent (Figure 2.6) [30].

But not only are humans affected: according to the IPCC, up to 30% of animal species will be at an increased risk of extinction by the middle of this century [13].

The following sections illustrate the changes in the environment that we are likely to experience with increasing frequency and intensity as temperatures continue to rise, and the effects these changes will have on health. The extent of these changes will depend on the rate and level of the mean annual temperature increase. Further details are available in the reports, publications and other sources for further information listed later in this chapter.

Heat waves

It is very important to make the distinction between *climate* and *weather*. Global climate changes are impossible for us to detect as individuals, and local weather events may give us the opposite – and wrong – impression. To give an example, although temperatures were unusually low in January 2010 in northern Europe and Asia, this month was one of the hottest on record globally, with some areas like the eastern Mediterranean and western Canada having been unusually warm [9]. It is important to look at long-term trends rather than the odd warm or cold month. Although global warming will lead to reduced energy demand for heating in some areas, the demand for cooling will increase in others.

Climate change will lead to more frequent and severe heat waves, which are periods of abnormally and uncomfortably hot and usually humid weather [31]. Many of the climate change models also predict dryer summers in the Northern hemisphere. The year 2010 was one of extremes in terms of heat [9]. On 26 July 2010, Moscow recorded its hottest day in 130 years, with a peak temperature of 37.5°C, only to be broken again a few days later, with a peak of 38.2°C. During the same year, temperatures soared to 52.5°C on 26 May 2010 in Pak Idan, and Pakistan logged its highest ever recorded temperature [9].

Severe heat waves lead to crop failures and water shortages, and may cause problems with energy supplies due to an increased use of electricity for air conditioning. Heat waves also carry the risk of people becoming seriously ill or dying from hyperthermia. Older people suffering from underlying cardiac or respiratory disease are particularly vulnerable, as the European heat wave in the summer of August 2003 has shown. According to an international team of epidemiologists, more than 70 000 excess deaths occurred as a direct result of the heat in Europe – the highest number of deaths from a heat wave ever recorded [32]. And in 1995, Chicago suffered from a heat wave that led to power failures which left thousands of people without electricity for up to two days [33]. Over 700 people died, making this heat wave one of the deadliest in American history. These striking examples vividly illustrate that high-income countries are not immune to the effects of global climate change. Of course, we cannot blame climate change alone, as various social, political and institutional factors also play a role in determining the effects of heat waves, particularly where they relate to inequalities [33].

It seems likely that later this century such hot periods will be the norm, rather than the exception [34]. Cities that already suffer from heat waves are likely to experience additional challenges through an increase in their number, duration and frequency this century [6]. However, it is also true that in colder areas, warmer winters would help protect certain vulnerable people, particularly older people and those with low income who suffer fuel poverty.

Extreme weather events and flooding

More frequent extreme weather as a result of global warming causes direct deaths from flooding and storms, which are already among the main causes of deadly types of natural disasters. Hurricanes, for example, develop when various factors come together. These include a sea surface temperature of at least 26.5°C (80°F), a temperature profile in the atmosphere that supports thunderstorm activity, sufficient water vapour in the in the troposphere and sufficient distance from the equator [35]. Even without understanding the intricacies of hurricane development, it is easy to realise how climate change can contribute to the development of severe weather and storms.

Some populations are likely to be more affected than others. Small island nations and low-income countries will be the first ones to be affected and suffer the hardest, particularly from drowning, injuries, communicable diseases and loss of livelihoods. Where vulnerable populations are affected, older people, children and those with underlying medical conditions will suffer the most [3, 6]. People in low-income countries suffering damage to their households or health are particularly vulnerable, as only about 1% of them are thought to have disaster insurance [36].

Analysis of long-term data shows a change in weather events, such as wind patterns and the intensity of tropical cyclones [13]. For example, westerly winds in mid-latitudes have become stronger in both hemispheres since the 1960s. Heavy rainfall has become more frequent over most land areas. And tropical cyclones in the North Atlantic and other areas have become more intense since the 1970s, although, so far, there is no clear trend indicating an increase in the yearly number of tropical storms. The IPCC predicts an increase in storms, leading to damage to housing and infrastructure [13]. Evidence suggests that in India and China this is already happening, in that heavy rainfall events are becoming heavier [37, 38]. In addition, two studies published in *Nature* directly link rising greenhouse gas levels with the growing intensity of rain and snow in the Northern Hemisphere [39, 40].

Extreme weather can be devastating. To give an example, in the same year that Pakistan experienced its highest recorded temperature, an active low pressure system moved south into the country, combining forces with the monsoon. As a result of the floods in July 2010, more than 18 million people suffered injuries and disease from polluted water, 1.7 million homes were damaged or destroyed and around 2000 people were killed [41].

Droughts and lack of freshwater supplies

Reliable access to clean drinking water and adequate sanitary conditions are important for people's health. But according to the WHO and UNICEF, two and a half billion people do not have access to adequate sanitation, which includes 1.2 billion people who have to defecate openly [42]. Almost 60% of people living in sub-Saharan Africa and Oceania do not have access to improved water facilities. Heat waves and altered weather patterns are likely to lead to further interruptions in freshwater supplies and reduced sanitation. Higher temperatures will also lead to water evaporating from the Earth's surface much faster and are already causing increased rates of melting in glaciers, which are important sources of fresh water in many areas. The IPCC estimates that between 75 and 250 million people will suffer increased water stress caused by climate change by the year 2020 [43]. Particularly in low-income countries, altered rainfall patterns and reduced supply from other sources (for example, because of disappearing glaciers) are likely to reduce the availability of drinking water as well as water needed for agriculture, energy generation and healthcare [6].

According to the IPCC, moist tropical areas and higher latitudes are likely to experience higher water availability, whereas areas that have lower annual rainfall will be exposed to reduced water availability and droughts [6]. In the next few decades, global agriculture will need to provide an increasing amount of food for emerging and growing economies. Recent models show that climate change, in addition to increases in water demands, changing water supplies and environmental flow requirements (that is, the quantity, timing and quality of water flows) required to sustain freshwater may lead to substantial a reduction in the availability of worldwide water for agriculture by 2050 (in the region of around 20%) [44]. The IPCC predicts that climate change will lead to changes in water quantity and quality, affecting food availability, access, stability and use [43].

Climate change can affect human health because it causes food insecurity and malnutrition, which are already prevalent, particularly so in many low-income countries [45]. According to the IPCC, smallholders, subsistence farmers and fishermen will suffer complex and localised negative impacts on food production [6]. Particularly in lower altitudes, cereal production is likely to decrease. Although in North America moderate climate change may increase aggregate rain-fed agricultural yields by an estimated 5–20%, crops that are sensitive to temperature increases or which are highly dependent on highly used water resources may suffer [6]. In addition to non-climate stressors, such as HIV, market failures and population increases, severe weather events are likely to damage crops and reduce yields from farming [46]. Results from six dynamic global vegetation models show that in four of the six models the net ecosystem productivity in tropical and southern hemisphere ecosystems is likely to decline after 2050 [47].

Sea level rise

Rising temperatures cause the thermal expansion of oceans and melting ice, which in turn lead to rising sea levels which threaten low-lying coastal communities around the world [13, 48, 49]. In the past century, mean sea levels rose by about 15 centimetres. Current trends suggest that we can expect a further rise of at least 18 centimetres by 2100 [49]. Uncertainty remains about the exact extent to which sea levels will rise. Conventional projections suggest a maximum rise of around 50 centimetres by 2100, but using different scenarios and taking into account the effects from melting ice in Antarctica and Greenland, levels in 2100 may be two metres higher than 1990. Even a rise in global mean sea level of one metre will have severe consequences for many coastal populations. For example, the Maldives and various island groups in the Pacific would almost certainly be largely inundated, and many coastal cities worldwide will be threatened [50]. But should large ice sheets such as those covering Greenland and Antarctica melt and collapse, sea levels might rise by another five metres. Although the probability of this happening over the next few centuries is low, global warming exceeding 2°C makes this – and the disastrous consequences – more likely.

Altered geographical distribution of insect vectors and communicable disease

A rise in global temperatures combined with altered patterns of rainfall and an increase in humidity is likely to cause a rise in infectious diseases by vectors, water and food. Some projections state that because of global climate change the number of people being at risk from malaria may increase by 90 million by the 2030 [51]. However, these figures may be lower, as claims that rising mean temperatures have already led to increases in malaria morbidity and mortality around the world are at odds with observations that malaria has, in fact, become less endemic and widespread, which suggests that any links of malaria distribution and climate are likely to also be affected by other factors [52].

For dengue fever, the expected increase would be even higher, with an estimated two billion people by the year 2080 [53]. From a combination of effects, we are likely to see a changed distribution and spreading of disease vectors, leading to an increased burden from diarrhoeal and other infectious diseases [6]. Outbreaks of diseases, such as cholera, will lead to an increase in morbidity and mortality from diarrhoeal disease, already amounting to around 1.8 million childhood deaths a year according to the WHO [3, 54].

Impact on global health inequalities, communities and migration

Wherever ecological or agricultural systems are impaired or destroyed, people's health will suffer directly. But there will also be indirect effects because of displacement and migration caused by civil conflict around space and resources. Having to leave a home or community behind can lead to a variety of health issues, including mental health problems and social isolation.

Increasing pressures on reduced natural resources also increases the risk of conflict and war between competing population groups [5]. Displacements and conflicts lead to cultural poverty and loss of identity, which may be difficult to measure but can have devastating effects on people's sense of wellbeing.

Although a changing climate will affect all of us, the health risks will vary depending on where people live, and under which circumstances [3]. For example, small islands and low-lying coastal regions are at particular risk from sea level rise, salinisation of water resources, floods and increasingly severe tropical storms. Combinations of heat waves, floods, infectious diseases or pollution affect urban populations – particularly those in very large tropical cities. For mountain populations, insecure water supplies, landslides and floods as well as infectious diseases will pose substantial health threats. Also, the health of populations living in polar regions (which are predicted to experience some of the world's greatest rises in average temperatures) may suffer disproportionately from climate change, affecting their food sources and thereby threatening their livelihoods.

Summary of the evidence and call to action

Knowing and understanding some of the key mechanisms and facts around environmental change and their implications for human health can help with appreciating the size and scale of the risks arising from these changes – and the consequences we face if we do not act fast. Looking at scientific evidence also brings home the fact that health services have a great opportunity to help mitigate, and adapt to, potentially very serious global environmental problems. The benefits of reducing greenhouse gas emissions and using non-renewable resources responsibly have never been clearer.

Although many actions that address climate change have clear financial, social and environmental benefits, it may be difficult to inspire or enact the changes needed to mitigate our risk. Similar to the classic grief reaction, learning more about this topic can make us sad, angry, guilty or ashamed. We will all have to be prepared to make changes in the way we live and work, some of which *appear* to be threatening, but many of which help us reassess what really determines a quality life. Modifying our behaviours can have many benefits (for example, we may become fitter and healthier by travelling more actively), but we may also feel a 'loss' if solutions cost money or impinge on currently perceived 'freedoms', such as driving a car or air travel.

To help us work through such painful emotions and even 'grief' that come with such changes, we need to gain at least a basic understanding of the key issues around climate change and health that will help us with changing our mindsets. And, of course, knowing about why and how climate change happens will help us to better engage with strategies for adaptation (which is managing the unavoidable) and mitigation (which is about avoiding the unmanageable).

Health professionals have important opportunities for pointing out these benefits to patients and policy makers. In the following chapters we describe the role that healthcare plays in the wider system and how we as health professionals, healthcare managers and policy makers can put theory into action. The next chapter gives a deeper insight into how people working in the health sector are part of a wider system and how changes that we make will affect other parts of this system.

Staying abreast with emerging evidence

Climate change research is a busy field. By the time this book is published, many new reports, research papers and recommendations will have come out. A list of resources that you may find useful for keeping abreast with new developments in the field of global environmental change and health is given in Box 2.1. Many of these resources contain links to other sources of information for anyone wishing to research a topic at a more detailed level.

Box 2.1 Resources for keeping up-to-date in the field of global environmental change and health

Key papers and reports

These key papers and reports are useful starting points for those looking for additional and more detailed information on the causes of global climate change and its impact on health:

Advancing the Science of Climate Research. National Research Council (2010). Available at www.americasclimatechoices.org

Climate Change: A Summary of the Science. The Royal Society (2010). Available at http://royalsociety.org/climate-change-summary-of-science/

Ecosystems and Human Well-Being: Health Synthesis from the Millennium Ecosystem Assessment. World Health Organization (2005). Available at http://www.who.int/globalchange/ecosystems/ecosys.pdf

Managing the health effects of climate change. Lancet and University College London Institute for Global Health Commission (2009). *Lancet*, **373**, 1693–1733.

IPCC Climate Change Fourth Assessment Report: Climate Change. United Nations Intergovernmental Panel on Climate Change (2007). Available at www.ipcc.ch/

Revision of Word Population Prospects. United Nations (2010). Available at www.un.org/en/development/progareas/population.shtml

Saving Carbon, Improving Health. NHS Carbon Reduction Strategy for England. NHS Sustainable Development Unit (2009). Available at www.sdu.nhs.uk/

Stern Review on the Economics of Climate Change (2006). Available at http://webarchive.nationalarchives.gov.uk/

Further information and staying up-to-date

In addition, the following organizations provide useful resources for keeping up with developments and trends in the field of global environmental change and health:

Berkeley Earth Surface Temperature, http://berkeleyearth.org/index.php

Center for Health and the Global Environment, Harvard Medical School, http://chge.med.harvard.edu/

Centers for Disease Control and Prevention (CDC), http://www.cdc.gov/climatechange/

Climate and Health Council, http://www.climateandhealth.org/

Global environmental change and human health project, www.essp.org

Health Care Without Harm, http://www.noharm.org/

Intergovernmental Panel on Climate Change (IPCC), http://www.ipcc.ch/

International Society of Doctors for the Environment, www.isde.org

Medact, http://www.medact.org/

NHS Sustainable Development Unit, www.sdu.nhs.uk/

Union of Concerned Scientists, http://www.ucsusa.org/ World Health Organization, www.who.int/globalchange/environment/en/

Key points

- Global climate change is caused by human activities.
- The impacts of climate change could increase exponentially.
- Global environmental change causes severe consequences for health.
- We still have time to avoid the worst impacts of climate change.
- Strong and early action outweighs the economic costs of not acting.
- The changes that we make in the next 10–20 years will affect the climate in the second half of this century and beyond – we need an international and immediate effort.

References

1. Costello, A., Abbas, M., Allen, A. *et al.* (2009) Managing the health effects of climate change. *Lancet*, **373** (9676), 1693–1733.
2. *The Economist* (2011) A new row about the IPCC: A climate of conflict [Internet]. Available from: http://www.economist.com/node/18866905 [accessed 17 July 2011].
3. World Health Organization (2008) *Protecting health from climate change: World Health Day 2008.* World Health Organization, Geneva, Switzerland.
4. Stern, N. (2007) *The economics of climate change : the Stern review.* Cambridge University Press, Cambridge.
5. World Economic Forum (2011) *Global Risks 2011*, 6th edn. World Economic Forum, Geneva, Switzerland.
6. Bernstein, L. (2008) *Climate change 2007: synthesis report. Intergovernmental Panel on Climate Change (IPCC)*, Geneva, Switzerland.
7. US National Research Council (2010) *Advancing the science of climate change: America's climate choices.* National Academies Press, Washington, DC.
8. Berkeley Earth Surface Temperature (Home) [Internet]. http://berkeleyearth.org/ [accessed 23 October 2011].
9. Met Office Hadley Centre (2011) Evidence: The state of the climate [Internet]. http://www.metoffice.gov.uk/media/pdf/m/6/evidence.pdf [accessed 31 July 2012).
10. Tans, P. and Keeling, R. – Trends in Carbon Dioxide [Internet]. http://www.esrl. noaa.gov/gmd/ccgg/trends/ [accessed June 2011].
11. Lüthi, D., Le Floch, M., Bereiter, B. *et al.* (2008) High-resolution carbon dioxide concentration record 650,000–800,000 years before present. *Nature*, **453**, 379–382.
12. OECD iLibrary – IEA CO2 Emissions from Fuel Combustion Statistics [Internet]. http://www.oecd-ilibrary.org/energy/data/iea-co2-emissions-from-fuel-combustion-statistics_co2-data-en [accessed 15 October 2011].
13. Solomon, S., Qin, D., Manning, M. *et al.* (2007) *Summary for Policy Makers. Climate Change 2007: The Physical Science Basis.* Contribution of Working

Group I to the Fourth Assessment Report of the Intergovernmental Panel on Climate Change. Cambridge University Press, Cambridge.

14. Trends in Carbon Dioxide [Internet]. http://www.esrl.noaa.gov/gmd/ccgg/trends/#mlo [accessed 23 October 2011].

15. Smith, K.R., Jerrett, M., Anderson, H.R. *et al.* (2010) Public health benefits of strategies to reduce greenhouse-gas emissions: health implications of short-lived greenhouse pollutants. *Lancet*, **374** (9707), 2091–2103.

16. Lovelock, J. (2009) *The Vanishing Face of Gaia: A Final Warning*. Allen Lane.

17. Winton, M. (2006) Amplified Arctic climate change: What does surface albedo feedback have to do with it? *Geophysical Research Letters* [Internet]. http://www.agu.org/pubs/crossref/2006/2005GL025244.shtml [accessed 15 October 2011].

18. Wickland, K.P., Striegl, R.G., Neff, J.C. and Sachs, T. (2006) Effects of permafrost melting on CO_2 and CH_4 exchange of a poorly drained black spruce lowland. *Journal of Geophysical Research* [Internet]. http://www.agu.org/pubs/crossref/2006/2005JG000099.shtml [accessed 15 October 2011].

19. The Royal Society (2010) *Climate change: A summary of the science*. The Royal Society, London.

20. Intergovernmental Panel on Climate Change (IPCC). Climate Change 2007: Synthesis Report. *Contribution of Working Groups I, II and III to the Fourth Assessment Report of the Intergovernmental Panel on Climate Change*. IPCC, Geneva, Switzerland. http://www.ipcc.ch/publications_and_data/publications_and_data_glossary.shtml [accessed 15 October 2011]

21. Lawson, N. (2009) *An Appeal to Reason: A Cool Look at Global Warming*. Gerald Duckworth and Co. Ltd, London.

22. Nilsson, M. (2009) Beaglehole R and Sauerborn R. *Climate policy: lessons from tobacco control. Lancet*, **374** (9706), 1955–1956.

23. Jacques, P.J., Dunlap, R.E. and Freeman, M. (2008) The organisation of denial: Conservative think tanks and environmental scepticism. *Environmental Politics*, **17** (3), 349–385.

24. Corvalaćn, C. (2005) Ecosystems and human well-being: health synthesis. *Millennium Ecosystem Assessment (Program)*, World Health Organization, Geneva, Switzerland.

25. United Nations (2005) *Living beyond our means: Natural assets and human well-being*. United Nations, New York.

26. Pretty, J. (2005) Countryside Recreation Network. *A countryside for health and wellbeing : the physical and mental health benefits of green exercise*. Countryside Recreation Network, Sheffield, UK.

27. Chivian, E. and Bernstein, A. (2008) *Sustaining Life: How Human Health Depends on Biodiversity*. OUP USA.

28. Hardin, G. (1968) The Tragedy of the Commons. *Science*, **162** (3859), 1243–1248.

29. Chan, M. (2007) Climate change and health: preparing for unprecedented challenges [Internet]. http://www.who.int/dg/speeches/2007/20071211_maryland/en/index.html [accessed 31 July 2011].

30. McMichael, A.J., Friel, S., Nyong, A. and Corvalan, C. (2008) Global environmental change and health: impacts, inequalities, and the health sector. *British Medical Journal*, **336** (7637), 191–194.

31. American Meteorological Society (2000) *The Glossary of Meteorology*. American Meteorological Society, Boston, MA.

32. Robine, J-M., Cheung, S.L.K., Le Roy, S. *et al.* (2008) Death toll exceeded 70,000 in Europe during the summer of 2003. *Comptes Rendus Biologies*, **331** (2), 171–178.

33. Klinenberg, E. (2002) *Heat Wave: A Social Autopsy of Disaster in Chicago*, 2nd edn. University of Chicago Press, IL.

34. Beniston, M. and Diaz, H. (2004) The 2003 heat wave as an example of summers in a greenhouse climate? Observations and climate model simulations for Basel, Switzerland. *Global and Planetary Change*, **44** (1–4), 73–81.

35. Hurricanes: Science and Society (University of Rhode Island) – Hurricane Genesis: Birth of a Hurricane [Internet]. http://www.hurricanescience.org/science/science/hurricanegenesis/ [accessed 15 October 2011].

36. Huq, S., Kovats, S., Reid, H. and Satterthwaite, D. (2007) Editorial: Reducing risks to cities from disasters and climate change. *Environment and Urbanization*, **19** (1), 3–15.

37. Dash, S.K., Kulkarni, M.A., Mohanty, U.C. and Prasad, K. (2009) Changes in the characteristics of rain events in India. *Journal of Geophysical Research* [Internet]. http://www.agu.org/pubs/crossref/2009/2008JD010572.shtml [accessed 22 July 2011].

38. Liu, B. (2005) Observed trends of precipitation amount, frequency, and intensity in China, 1960–2000. *Journal of Geophysical Research* [Internet]. http://www.agu.org/pubs/crossref/2005/2004JD004864.shtml [accessed 22 July 2011].

39. Min, S-K., Zhang, X., Zwiers, F.W. and Hegerl, G.C. (2011) Human contribution to more-intense precipitation extremes. *Nature*, **470**, 378–381.

40. Pall, P., Aina, T., Stone, D.A. *et al.* (2011) Anthropogenic greenhouse gas contribution to flood risk in England and Wales in autumn 2000. *Nature*, **470**, 382–385.

41. Scott, M. (2011) Heavy Rains and Dry Lands Don't Mix: Reflections on the 2010 Pakistan Flood : [Internet]. http://earthobservatory.nasa.gov/Features/PakistanFloods/printall.php [accessed 6 December 2011].

42. World Health Organization/UNICEF. Progress on sanitation and drinking-water: 2010 *update*. WHO/UNICEF, Geneva, Switzerland. 2010.

43. Bates, B. (2008) *Intergovernmental Panel on Climate Change*. Climate change and water technical paper of the Intergovernmental Panel on Climate Change. Intergovernmental Panel on Climate Change, Geneva, Switzerland.

44. Strzepek, K. and Boehlert, B. (2010) Competition for water for the food system. *Philosophical Transactions of the Royal Society B: Biological Sciences*, **365** (1554), 2927–2940.

45. Brown, M.E. and Funk, C.C. (2008) CLIMATE: Food Security Under Climate Change. *Science*, **319** (5863), 580–581.

46. Morton, J.F. (2007) Climate Change and Food Security Special Feature: The impact of climate change on smallholder and subsistence agriculture. *Proceedings of the National Academy of Sciences USA*, **104** (50), 19680–19685.

47. Cramer, W., Bondeau, A., Woodward, F.I. *et al.* (2001) Global response of terrestrial ecosystem structure and function to CO_2 and climate change: results from six dynamic global vegetation models. *Global Change Biology*, **7** (4), 357–373.

48. Intergovernmental Panel on Climate Change (2007) *The Physical Science Basis: Working Group I Contribution to the Fourth Assessment Report of the IPCC*, 1st edn. Cambridge University Press.

49. Vermeer, M. and Rahmstorf, S. (2009) Global sea level linked to global temperature. *Proceedings of the National Academy of Sciences USA*, **106** (51), 21527–21532.

50. Dow, K. and Downing, T.E. (2011) *The Atlas of Climate Change*, 3rd edn. Routledge.

51. Hay, S., Tatem, A., Guerra, C. and Snow, R. (2006) Foresight on population at malaria risk in Africa: 2005, 2015 and 2030. *Scenario review paper prepared for the Detection and Identification of Infectious Diseases Project (DIID)*. Forsight Project, Office of Science and Innovation, London.

52. Gething, P.W., Smith, D.L., Patil, A.P., Tatem, A.J., Snow, R.W. and Hay, S.I. (2010) Climate change and the global malaria recession. *Nature*, **465**, 342–345.

53. Hales, S., deWet, N., Maindonald, J. and Woodward, A. (2002) Potential effect of population and climate changes on global distribution of dengue fever: an empirical model. *Lancet*, **360** (9336), 830–834.

54. Black, R.E., Allen, L.H., Bhutta, Z.A. *et al.* (2008) Maternal and child undernutrition: global and regional exposures and health consequences. *Lancet*, **371** (9608), 243–260.

Chapter 3 **Engaging with sustainability**

In this chapter

- What is sustainability?
- Learning from systems thinking
- Resilience in human health
- Climate change denial explored
- Engaging with the earth system
- Useful terms and concepts in sustainability

The situation of the Earth system in the *Anthropocene* is perilous, as we have mapped out in the first two chapters. Healthcare is both part of the problem and part of the solution, and in Chapters 5 to 12 of this book we look at the practical things that people working in the sector can do to address the massive problems ahead. This chapter is designed to broaden and deepen our understanding of sustainability beyond basic meanings and metrics. To do this we will draw particularly on the insights of *systems theory*, a branch of knowledge which has been applied across diverse areas, such as management, family therapy and engineering. We consider the Earth as a vast and arguably living system, and give particular attention to the foundational concept of *resilience*, which has particular resonance in the health field.

People are becoming increasingly aware of the ecological issues of our times; yet reflecting that awareness in how we act in the world can be tough, even for the most committed. In this chapter we introduce the idea of *carbon dependency* and draw on models from the addictions field to explore this dissonance. For overcoming carbon addiction and engaging practically with our predicaments, this chapter seeks inspiration from ancient myth, traditional culture and contemporary poetry. We close with a look at some of the major concepts of sustainability, such as *carbon footprinting* and *virtuous cycles*. As a first step we explore what sustainability means as an overarching idea.

Sustainable Healthcare, First Edition. Knut Schroeder, Trevor Thompson, Kathleen Frith and David Pencheon.
© 2013 John Wiley & Sons, Ltd. Published 2013 by John Wiley & Sons, Ltd.

The sustainable picnic

If I buy that house, will those mortgage repayments be sustainable or leave me financially stretched? Are the fostering arrangements for that disturbed child sustainable or likely to breakdown with their next violent outburst? Is that new urban hospital sustainable or likely to run out of patients as care shifts to the community? Our general sense of sustainability is as a measure of the long-term viability of a thing or process. In 1987, a United Nations commission helpfully extended the concept by defining sustainable development as meeting 'the needs of the present without compromising the ability of future generations to meet their own needs' [1]. Imagine a picnic. You go to the beach and have a leisurely lunch. When it is time to go most people intuitively feel the need to clear up all their rubbish and put it in a bin or take it home. We do not like coming to a beach covered in refuse and so we do not leave the place looking like a tip for the next party. It does not take much ethical imagination to understand this principle, and few would contest it. Yet it is clearly one the human community has struggled to put into practice. Sticking with the seaside, consider how some marine ecologies have been so exploited that biologists believe they will never recover. The once abundant Newfoundland cod, for example, feeds on smaller fish and crustaceans that themselves feed on cod larvae. With the collapse of adult cod stocks through over-fishing, the population of these predators has expanded so much that cod larvae numbers are perpetually suppressed [2]. This is a clear example of how present actions foreclose on future possibilities. To gain a more nuanced understanding of sustainability we must consider not only desirable outcomes (like plenty of cod) but also the internal processes that make those outcomes likely. For this we turn now to the insights of systems theory.

Understanding systems

The medical community is used to talking about systems, such as the cardiovascular system, the respiratory system or the immune system. It is curious that medical education does not typically involve teaching about systems *in general*: what systems are, how they tend to behave and how they can go wrong [3]. To address this need, the University of Bristol has introduced a lecture on *systems thinking* for medical students; it is co-presented by a clinician and a medical physiologist. Physiological systems provide particularly clear examples of system behaviour, exemplified in the following sections, which introduce the basic ideas.

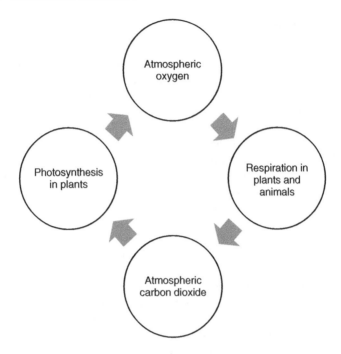

Figure 3.1 The oxygen cycle.

Open and cyclical systems

An open system is one that exchanges things with its surroundings. It has *inflows* and it has *outflows*. In textbooks, systems are, for simplicity, often represented *as if* they are closed, when in fact they are open. Take the respiratory system as an example. It is an enlightened respiratory physiologist who pays homage to plants in their lectures, as without plants there is no oxygen to inspire and no processing of expired carbon dioxide. So the lungs are part of an open system which includes the rainforest, and it is curious how in this regard we talk of the respiratory 'tree'. Sustainability is about preserving our inputs (resources) and ensuring the safe disposal of our outputs (waste). Often in nature, the outflows of one system form the inflows of another to create a *cycle*. Think, for instance, of the relationship between photosynthesis and tissue respiration in the oxygen cycle (Figure 3.1).

Expect trouble when humans dislocate these natural cycles. For instance, the *Three Gorges Dam* on China's Yangtze River produces carbon-free hydroelectric power and reduces the risk of seasonal flooding. But the vast concrete barrier also prevents the annual seaward migration of 530 million tonnes of sediment – sediment that once reinforced the foundations of the mega-city of Shanghai, but which is now accumulating in the 40 km^3 reservoir [4]. To think sustainably, then, is to think *cyclically*. For instance, how we relate as a culture to the return of the dead human body to elemental cycles has major sustainability implications, as we explore in Chapter 10.

The (often hidden) parts in networks

The constituent parts of systems are often not evident. When we ask students to draw a tree, about 90% draw a tree without roots. But a tree without roots is, of course, not really a tree at all (Figure 3.2).

This insight then leads to a discussion of what bits are prone to be 'missing' from the everyday medical understanding of the sick person from a systems point of view. Answers include the family, the subconscious, the patient's emotional state, their personal 'story' and issues like stigma and discrimination. In the planetary system, atmospheric gases, being invisible, are also easily overlooked. Were we able to actually *see* carbon dioxide, our

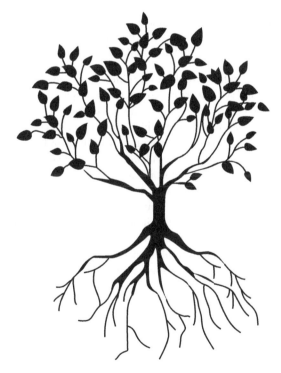

Figure 3.2 A tree is incomplete without roots. (Reproduced with permission from www.featurepics.com, Image # 13158503 copyright ©Olivier26.)

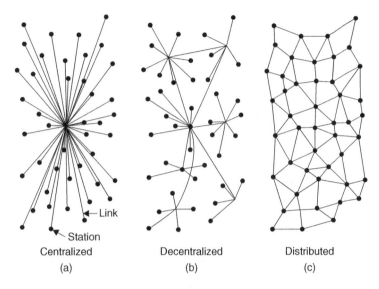

Centralized   Decentralized   Distributed
(a)   (b)   (c)

Figure 3.3 Centralised, decentralised and distributed networks. (Reproduced with permission by the RAND corporation, available at http://www.rand.org/pubs/research_memoranda/RM3420.html.)

attitude to it as a substance would be very different. To complicate matters, the parts of real-world systems are not connected in simple linear arrangements. For instance, members of a community are connected in complex webs known as social networks, a term which predates the internet era [5]. As a consequence, the health of a system is often determined by the quality of such connections. For instance, in the *Alameda County Study*, the age-adjusted relative risks of death for the most isolated participants compared to those with the most social contacts were 2.3 for men and 2.8 for women [6]. This association held even after adjusting for other usual determinants of longevity, such as smoking. The way in which parts are networked has major implications for system performance. Figure 3.3a shows a centralized network in which information is shared only with a central control point – the pattern most favoured by dictators and despots. Sustainable systems are more likely to be decentralized (Figure 3.3b) or distributed (Figure 3.3c). The reason these networks function differently can be understood with another fundamental aspect of system behaviour – feedback.

Feedback loops

Connections between parts of systems comprise two types of feedback loops: *normative* and *amplificatory*. Normative loops are responsible for keeping things stable. As the level of a parameter rises, the normative loop acts to bring it down again. Normative loops control physiological parameters, such as blood pressure, glucose levels, posture and appetite. A healthy normative loop responds with sensitivity to changes in the external and internal environment. Studies have, for instance, shown that cardiac patients with more variable heart rates live longer than those with more constant heart rates [7]. If these normative loops are too reactive, then the system can become brittle, unable to experiment or 'play'. But where a system does not adequately respond to normative feedback signals, the parameter in question can spiral out of control. In higher organisms, cancer cells show this tendency. When healthy cells meet, they stop growing through 'contact inhibition', but cancer cells continue to replicate and pile up on top of each other. In the context of the global system, climate change signals distress (Chapters 1 and 2), yet humanity continues to produce increasing amounts of carbon dioxide, risking catastrophic global warming – a clear failure of a normative loop.

The second type of feedback mechanism is the *amplificatory* loop, which acts the opposite way. In amplificatory loops, the output of the system *enhances* its own production. Physiological examples include orgasm, ovulation and childbirth. For instance, when the cervix (the neck of the womb) stretches during childbirth, the pituitary gland at the base of the brain releases the hormone oxytocin. This hormone helps the uterus to contract, which in turn stretches the cervix further, producing even more oxytocin in the brain. This amplificatory process continues until the baby is born. Natural amplificatory loops apply to time-limited processes, as things in nature do not amplify indefinitely. But for people and the planet, amplificatory loops can be pathological if the parameter in question is not desirable and amplifies out-of-control. Ice-melts at high latitudes due to global warming provide a good example. As seawater replaces the polar ice, less light is reflected and more heat is absorbed, consequently leading to higher water temperatures and even more melting ice. These are sometimes called *runaway* effects, which end with the system finding a different, and potentially detrimental, resting equilibrium. Learning to identify the presence and influence of normative and amplificatory feedback loops is an important step in creating and maintaining sustainable systems.

Emergence, self-organisation and coherence

While ideas around feedback loops are fairly well known, the concept of *emergence* may not be so familiar. Emergence is an established scientific phenomenon in which system components, through simple interactions, spontaneously assemble themselves into much more complex formations that 'emerge' without any central controlling element [8]. Think, for instance, of the unique geometry of snowflakes, each formed from the same water molecules, or the complex behaviour of social insects such as termites, which industriously construct complex air-conditioned mounds, each insect acting without an overall awareness of the grand design [9]. Living systems, unlike purely mechanical entities, have an inherent tendency to take on an orderly structure and function, which has been termed *self-organisation* [10]. Another important concept is *coherence*, which describes how parts work synergistically to achieve the purpose of the system, without any overt lines of control. In everyday life, coherence corresponds to the elusive 'zone' in sport or 'flow' in musical performance. The idea that systems have an intrinsic coherence has major medical and sustainability implications, as we shall see.

Earth as a system

Complex systems have the remarkable capacity to self-regulate. As we know, the human body, for example, maintains physiological parameters, such as blood glucose, within a narrow reference range, and does this consistently across all humans. A complex buffering mechanism, for instance, keeps the blood pH in healthy people stable between 7.35 and 7.45. This same ability to self-regulate exists for the Earth as a whole; the evidence for such self-regulation is very strong [11]. *Gaia Theory* (from the Greek 'gaia', meaning 'Earth' or 'goddess of the Earth'), first hypothesised in 1974 by the climatologist James Lovelock, proposes that all organisms and their inorganic surroundings on Earth are closely integrated to form a single and self-regulating complex system which maintains the conditions for life on the planet [12]. For instance, we know from ice-core data that concentrations of atmospheric oxygen, carbon dioxide and methane have remained stable over several hundred thousand years at levels that are critical for maintaining life. According to Gaia Theory, this constancy does not happen by chance but is due to the interplay of living organisms with the 'inorganic' atmosphere, actively maintaining gases at these levels. For instance, as atmospheric carbon dioxide rises, more is photosynthesised by algae in the oceans into sugars and oxygen in a simple normative feedback loop. Similar mechanisms exist to maintain the Earth's temperature and the salinity of the oceans. This is analogous to what we know of human homeostasis and has caused some to consider the Earth as a living organism. Just like we take abnormal blood test results as signs of systemic upset, so we know that rising levels of atmospheric carbon dioxide (currently the highest for at least 800 000 years) are signs of global stress. The capacity of the Earth system to buffer carbon dioxide (and hence global temperature) is reaching its limit. Though the idea of the Earth as a self-regulating system is now widely accepted within Earth Sciences, its implications are only beginning to unravel [12]. For instance, Lovelock holds the view that gradual climate change, as modelled by the *Intergovernmental Panel on Climate Change (IPCC)* (Chapter 2) is unlikely and that according to Gaia Theory the Earth may shift rapidly into a 'hot state', with a restricted biosphere [13].

So far we have looked at some important systems properties, such as the open system, cyclicity, hidden parts, networks and emergence, with Gaia Theory as a global exemplar. But from a health perspective, one systems concept is of especial value, and that is the idea of *resilience*.

Resilience in health

When we ask people 'What is health?', they might offer us the WHO definition of health as 'a state of complete physical, mental and social wellbeing and not merely the absence of disease or infirmity' (1946). Although this explanation widens our definitional scope, it does not explore the 'how' behind the 'what' of health, so suffers the same limitations as conventional definitions of sustainability. This definition also sets an absolute standard of health that makes it practically unobtainable, given our aging population and the prevalence of long-term conditions. It is heartening, then, to read of new international initiatives to rework the WHO definition towards concepts of *resilience, adaption* and *self-management* [14]. The examples given in Case study 3.1 illustrate the concept of resilience in an inner-city setting.

These case studies form a starting point for exploring the idea of *resilience*, defined by the Oxford English Dictionary as 'the quality or fact of being able to recover quickly or easily from, or resist being affected by, a misfortune, shock, illness, etc.'[16]. Researchers have found three factors that predict resilience: *individual* attributes (such as an engaging 'easy' temperament), *relational* attributes (for example, parental relationships with high trust, warmth and cohesion) and *external support systems* (good neighbourhoods and schools, for instance) [17]. This modelling rings true for Patsy and Ayana. Ayana is blessed with an engaging temperament; she grew up with strong family ties that she has maintained into adulthood, and she is well integrated within the Bristol Somali community. Patsy, on the other hand, has a fractious and pleading temperament that does not invite engagement. She has experienced poor parenting and has limited and troubled contact with her own children. Her only social interactions are the statutory services and a kindly neighbour.

The concept of resilience also applies to much larger scales of organisation. Ecologists talk of the resilience of whole ecosystems to threats such as fire, flood and exploding insect populations [18]. They describe the idea of *latitude*, which is the extent to which we can push a system before it changes

Case study 3.1   Resilience in an inner-city setting (Based on Resilience studies from the practice of Dr Trevor Thompson [15])

We see a lot of Patsy*. She requests home visits from the Primary Care Team about once every two weeks. She complains of abdominal pain that has been extensively investigated without a biomedical cause being found. She feels depressed, does not respond to antidepressants and is unmoved by reassurance. She is estranged from her daughters. She smokes heavily and takes five prescription medications. The best efforts of our team have yet to trigger a shift in her health and health-seeking behaviour, though we continue to try. Her commonest complaint is that she cannot cope. She seeks help from us but struggles to articulate exactly what it is that would make a difference.

I got to know Ayana* over several years. She consults infrequently, mainly with her children. She came to the United Kingdom from The Netherlands in 2003. She fled to The Netherlands from war-torn Somalia. She is a tall, elegant woman with a flashing smile. After our last consultation, I asked the student with me at the time if she had noticed anything unusual. The student commented on the high standard of her English but had not noticed her left hand which was missing three fingers. Ayana had been hit, aged 13, by a random mortar round that had killed her sister and mother as they sat cooking in their compound in Mogadishu. I once treated Ayana for headaches and got to hear her story. She felt no bitterness, she focused her life on her family and her community, she attends evening classes and is about to obtain bookkeeping qualifications.

Patsy and Ayana live in the same high-rise block in inner city Bristol but it is hard to imagine two people more differently situated in the world. Both have been forced to cope with great adversity (Patsy's father was an alcoholic), and who is to say who has suffered more? But presently one is dependent, isolated and unhappy, and the other is independent, well connected – and the sort of person you feel better for spending time with.

*names changed to preserve anonymity

Extract reproduced from [15] Thompson T. Resilience – a concept comes of age. Journal of Holistic Healthcare. 2011;8(2):19–22.

beyond the point of (easy) recovery to its original state. Many will remember their disappointment as a child when their 'slinky' (a long sprung metal coil) became overstretched and would no longer perform its usual tricks. Living systems risk a similar fate. In a medical context, think metastatic cancer or psychotic breakdown. It takes a great act of faith to imagine Patsy functioning as a wholesome independent citizen. Somewhere along the line she appears to have passed the 'point of no return'. Another useful concept is that of *precariousness*, which describes a system that is working close to its point of maximum latitude. Although a precarious system *appears* to be functioning normally, it is prone to breakdown when confronted by relatively trivial stress – the 'straw that breaks the camel's back'. Increasing evidence suggests that the global ecosystem is likely to be at just such a point.

Promoting resilience

Promoting resilience is a central purpose of healthcare. In a resilient system, the parts are well connected through responsive feedback loops. If there was one scale upon which Patsy and Ayana could be most distinctly compared, it would be *connectedness*. Connectedness can relate to friends, family and neighbours, and also internally between, for instance, instinct and reason. Consequently, the quality and quantity of community ties consistently correlate with proxy measures of health [6, 19]. Resilience can also be affected by the use of pharmaceuticals. From a purely medical perspective, we can be grateful for the range of drugs and surgical interventions that modern medicine has to offer. But by removing feedback signals (such as indigestion, fatigue or headache), medication can deprive the body of the information it needs to re-establish its internal regulation, for example by motivating a needed lifestyle modification. Taking medication externalises both the problem and the solution, so making pharmaceuticals the fulcrum of medical care may not be the best route to a sustainable system.

Resilient systems are usually *diverse* systems. It makes intuitive sense that the wider the range of resources a system can call upon, the more likely it is to survive and thrive [20]. For instance, agricultural monocultures (farming dependent on a single crop) are vulnerable to pestilence and climate vagaries, whereas diverse systems find it easier to adapt [21]. There are many similar analogies in the field of health. For example, health systems need diversity in sourcing energy to reduce fossil fuel dependence [22], practitioners need diversity in their medical models in case any one model proves limited and, as individuals, we need a diversity of ways to get and stay healthy, which may well include interventions that are still outside the conventional canon.

Resilient systems also show *redundancy*, an attribute that has positive connotations in the systems context. Redundancy as an idea means that the system has non-active elements that it can quickly activate as and when the need arises. This idea is not only key to engineering where system failure can be catastrophic (think reserve parachutes) but also relates to the idea of *social capital* [23], a term that describes the reserves of social connectedness upon which we can draw in times of trouble.

Thus far we have considered sustainability in systems terms and placed in the foreground the idea of resilience as a key concept for the future. We have looked at connectedness, diversity and redundancy as system characteristics that promote such resilience. Throughout the book we will clothe these concepts with further examples. Having unpacked the idea of sustainability in a systems context, we now look at how we can engage with it – as individuals and as agents of change.

Gauging engagement

In 2009, the World Bank published the results of an international survey on public attitudes to climate change; the survey was conducted by a team from the University of Maryland [24]. This study showed that, on average, 59% of citizens considered climate change to be a very *serious* problem, with even higher percentages in low-income countries. But climate change collides with other competing concerns. For instance, US citizens were asked in May 2010 by the pollsters *Gallup* what they considered to be the *most important* problems currently facing their country. The environment was cited by only 3% of respondents, behind the economy, jobs, healthcare costs, immigration and terrorism [25]. People increasingly engage with sustainability issues, but the overall level of engagement remains limited. Most people still lack an awareness of the issues, but even those who are well informed and care passionately about the situation of the Earth still have difficulty changing their behaviours and lining them up with their values. We are all creatures of habit, and habits are notoriously difficult to shift. At the extreme end of the spectrum we have those damaging and inveterate habits we term *addictions*.

Carbon dependence syndrome

Frances Mortimer and the UK's *Centre for Sustainable Healthcare* have developed the concept of 'carbon dependence syndrome' (CDS) as a tongue-in-cheek and yet plausibly reasoned metaphor for our current 'addiction' to high-carbon lifestyles (www.carbonaddict.org). In its early stages, an addictive behaviour can bring much pleasure, but as it develops people feel powerless to resist in the face of significant negative consequences. Fossil fuels have fuelled a lot of pleasure in recent history. We love our cars, our

Box 3.1   Carbon Dependency Syndrome CAGE Questionnaire

Have you ever felt you should Cut your carbon use (electricity / travel / meat intake / shopping)?:	YES/NO
Have people ever Annoyed you by criticizing your carbon use?:	YES/NO
Have you ever felt bad or Guilty about your carbon footprint?:	YES/NO
Have you ever had a fix*first thing in the morning to steady your nerves? (Eye-opener):	YES/NO

*Some examples of a carbon fix: >15-min shower / morning car commute / bacon and sausage breakfast / early bout of internet shopping (reproduced, with permission, from www.carbonaddict.org).

If you have two or more 'YES' responses you may be living with Carbon Dependency Syndrome.

flights, our gadgets, our warm houses, our convenient and plentiful food. But have we also become dependent on these things just to feel 'OK'? We can now self-diagnose CDS by using a modification of the CAGE questionnaire used in the diagnosis of alcoholism (Box 3.1) [26].

Of course, the pangs of addiction are most keenly felt only when we stop consuming, which in the case of CDS we rarely do. The negative consequences of the above are not just for *Gaia*, but writ large in heart disease, obesity, diabetes and mental health problems. A valuable consequence of seeing our carbon use as an addiction is that it allows us to apply the accumulated wisdom from the field of addiction treatment. Most clinicians will be familiar with the *stages of change model* by Proschaska and DiClemente (Figure 3.4) [27].

This model segments the process of change based on the idea that people at different stages respond differently to interventions. Clinicians will recognise the fruitlessness of berating the pre-contemplative smoker with a litany of facts about the dangers of tobacco. Similarly, the person who is preparing to reduce their carbon use will welcome specific advice on low-carbon living more than exhortations on the perils of climate change. Additionally, is it good to know that relapse is a normal part of the addiction cycle; successful quitters often succeed after multiple attempts and moving on from relapse is a key skill, at a time when self-esteem may be faltering. For instance, a person committed to carbon reduction may question the worth of *all* their efforts after booking a long-haul flight. For those wanting to be agents for change

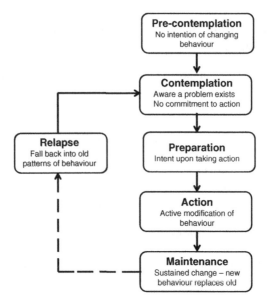

Figure 3.4 The stages of change model. (Adapted from Proschaska and DiClemente [27].)

in the addictions field there is one posture that it is particularly important to understand – and that is *denial*.

Dissecting denial

Coming to terms with new and uncomfortable information is difficult for everyone. For instance, a patient diagnosed with a malignancy will often doubt or deny their diagnosis, as frank disbelief is recognised as part of the grieving process [28]. While healthy scepticism plays an important part in critically assessing the predictions of climate scientists, outright denial of climate change is best understood as a psychological coping strategy. According to addictions specialist Dr Chris Johnson, denial of our pending environmental crisis has the same features as denial found in the general addictions field. It is part of a process of coming to terms with something initially too uncomfortable to accept [29]. That these issues are global paradoxically makes them easier to ignore, because the problem and the solution can easily feel remote. If the call to a low-carbon lifestyle threatens possessions and activities that we hold dear (cars or long-haul flights, for instance), then we can compartmentalise our response by engaging in (possibly tokenistic) green behaviours such as recycling, while still driving a car more than we really need to, or jetting about the world on a regular basis. Changing our behaviours is a complex process as we try and reconcile such conflicting urges. For example, we might want to lose weight, but also really love the experience of eating chocolate. Activists such as Joanna Macy have learned to focus more on listening to people's responses than assaulting them with doom-laden information, preferring unpacking to paralysis [30]. The carbon-dependent person, unlike someone with severe alcohol problems, may not readily feel the harms of their addiction. For affluent and physically healthy people to adopt a low-carbon lifestyle, they will need to draw on motivations deeper than their immediate and personal wellbeing. In the following section we highlight different sources of such inspiration.

Connecting with the Earth system

Most of us have a particular place to which we return either in person or in our memories that helps us maintain a strong sense of connection to landscape or nature. Not uncommonly this is a place from childhood, such as a mountain, a beach or a forest. This *connection* is not a reasoned response, but a feeling perhaps of wonder, peace or gratitude. We are now starting to understand how important these connections are for regulating our emotions [31], and threats to these personal myths can trigger strong ecological motivation. One of us (TT) spent an idyllic childhood summer around the English village of Chelsfield, just south of London. Returning twenty years later he was viscerally stunned to discover six roaring lanes of the M25 London orbital motorway careering over the same fields.

Such personal stories resonate with those of an animate Earth documented in humanity's mythological traditions, where the Earth is often referred to as a goddess – though certainly not always a wholly kind one. In very recent memory we have seen the devastation enacted by natural forces such as floods, tsunamis, droughts and earthquakes. The Earth, or *Gaia*, as a self-regulating entity may not have the survival of humanity as a prime concern. She might just as well be named *Nemesis* or *Kali*. Perhaps this is why humanity has focused so much on her domination. From a systems perspective, the notion of the 'conquest' of nature seems absurd. This is a metaphor used by Francis Bacon (1561–1626), Enlightenment scholar and recognised founder of the modern scientific method. Bacon said, 'we shall perhaps at last learn the noblest lesson of all, that man must not fight man, but must make war only on the obstacles that nature offers to the triumph of man' [32]. This bold vision predicts the extraordinary technological achievements of humankind for which we are rightly grateful. But it is also a difficult cultural heritage from which to forge a new affective relationship with the Earth system.

From traditional cultures we have insights from peoples who have lived over millennia in close relation to the Earth. Australian Aborigines [33], Kalahari Bushmen [34], and the native North American Indians [35] have given us many insights about how the Earth functions as a system. In healthcare, traditional medical systems like Ayurvedic and Chinese medicine perceive the world comprised of interacting elements, such as wood, metal, fire and water. The purpose of medicine in these traditional systems is to promote harmony between these elements in the person and in their environment in an elegant exposition of systems thinking that can inform our design in contemporary healthcare [36].

Poets speak the harder truths of our predicament in poems of reverence, hope, consternation and despair. Here is what might now be called an 'ecopoem' by the Irish poet Brendan Kennelly (b 1936) from Neil Astley's collection 'Earth Shattering' [37]:

The Hope of Wings
The girl forces the gull's beak open with
A spoon and starts to scrape the oil away.
Rampant the sky's colours, legend and myth
Sustain the attention of those beset by
Traditional hungers, but now I foresee
A bird-emptied sky, the world's shores
Hilled with crippled things, the thick, black
Smothering oil murdering the hope of wings.
And this girl – she can't be into her teens –
Would, if her working now is a guide,
Spend all her years remaking these stunned birds
Littering the sea, dead flops among stones.
She'd give a white-winged creature to the sky
Before black tides drown mere human words.

Brendan Kennelly (b 1936)
Reproduced with permission from [37] 'The Hope of Wings' from
Brendan Kennelly, Familiar Strangers: New and Selected Poems
1960–2004. Bloodaxe Books Ltd; 2004.

Such poetry is a strong way to help people begin to engage, with hearts as well as heads. Connecting with the Earth system may seem a long way from the conventional and often frantic clinical front line. But the deeper our connection to the natural world, the more likely we are to engage in practical action.

A lexicon of sustainability

Like medicine, the field of sustainability has its own 'language' with terms that will emerge repeatedly in the following chapters. In the following sections we define some of the most important.

Virtuous cycles

We have already met amplificatory feedback loops in our discussion of systems theory. *Virtuous cycles* are types of feedback loops in which change in one domain benefits other domains, both locally and systemically. In the sustainability context, we often use this phrase to describe behavioural changes that are of simultaneous benefit to both people and the environment. For instance, people who cycle to work rather than hop in the car and drive, protect their hearts, better their moods, improve the local environment and reduce carbon emissions – while saving money into the bargain. These benefits are also referred to as health *co-benefits* [38]. The existence of such virtuous cycles is not just a happy accident but implies coherence.

Mitigation and adaptation

Mitigation (of climate change) is about actions to *reduce* the quantities of greenhouse gases in the atmosphere and, hence, global warming. In healthcare terms, this is akin to primary prevention. This can be achieved, for example, through reducing demand for carbon-intensive commodities, investing in renewables and improving the efficiency of essential services like healthcare, transport, lighting, cooking and heating. Alternatively, we can achieve mitigation through technologies that retrieve carbon dioxide from the atmosphere and move it into carbon sinks. Such mitigation may slow the current rate of global warming (which would continue even if all carbon emissions ceased today). *Adaptation* is about societal activities that help us *adjust* to the facts of climate change. Examples of adaptation include creating flood defences, preparing for climate change-induced migration and developing a drought-resistant agriculture. Commentators such as James Lovelock argue that catastrophic climate change is almost inevitable, so that we should now be focusing mainly on adaptation – even if only to buy time for mitigation [13].

Contraction and convergence

Contraction is straightforward to understand, if far from straightforward to implement. The world community sets national carbon quotas to gradually *contract* people's carbon dioxide emissions to a sustainable level, currently estimated at two tonnes of carbon dioxide per year for each citizen of the world, which is around 13% of the current United Kingdom and 7% of the United States emissions per person. This target aims to keep carbon dioxide concentrations at less than 450 ppm (Chapter 2) and global warming at less than two degrees Celsius. This, as we know, will come with substantive health co-benefits as we swop motorcars for muscle. *Convergence* recognises that currently many poor nations actually create *less* carbon than the two-tonnes-per-person-per-year target. Under a convergence scheme, these countries could either increase their industrial capacity or sell their carbon entitlement to the rich world through carbon trading schemes.

Carbon literacy and numeracy

Many of us have a good sense of what things cost, such as going out for a meal, buying a new laptop computer or insuring a car. We have this sense because we make purchasing decisions in relation to our income. Spending more than we earn brings trouble in the long term. What most of us do not have is a similar sense of the *carbon* costs of our common activities and acquisitions. And this is because we, societally, have never considered carbon as a commodity that we need to control. There are currently no limits to the amount of carbon we are *personally* responsible for releasing into the skies. Yet there is compelling evidence that, like with fiscal debt, we are storing trouble for our collective futures through anthropogenic climate change. If we each had annual carbon budgets, just like we have annual monetary incomes, we would, of course, rapidly develop the necessary carbon literacy and numeracy to balance the books. In the meantime, what can we do to start to get a feel for the carbon costs of modern life?

All global citizens should commit certain carbon numerals to memory, such as the current parts per million of atmospheric carbon dioxide (394 ppm in March 2012) [39]. Another is the average *carbon footprint* of persons in different countries. The carbon footprint is a measure of the amount of greenhouse gases produced through burning fossil fuels for commodity manufacture, electricity, heating, transport and so on. It is measured in units of kilograms or metric tonnes (1000 kg) of carbon dioxide equivalents (CO_2e). The CO_2e concept takes account of the fact that there are various greenhouse gases (GHGs) in the atmosphere, such as methane and nitrogen dioxide, with differing potentials to cause global warming. The impact of these different gases is measured in relation to carbon dioxide, to create the composite unit of CO_2e. Individuals, groups and even whole organisations can estimate their carbon footprint by using online carbon calculators, such as the one available at www.carbonfootprint.com. However, these calculators

Table 3.1   Carbon dioxide equivalents (CO_2e) emissions by country per person per year (2009 figures) [41].

Country	CO_2e (in metric tonnes) per person per annum
Bangladesh	1.1
Brazil	4.1
China	3.1
Germany	15.1
India	1.8
Uganda	1.1
United Kingdom	15.4
United States	28.6

can systematically underestimate carbon emissions by focusing on home energy and transport, so it is important to also account for consumer products such as food and electrical goods [40]. Hertwich and Peters have produced a rigorous analysis of CO_2e calculations by nation, taking into account the consumption of imported goods (it would, for instance, be wrong to attribute carbon emissions for manufactured goods to China when, in fact, these goods are being consumed in Europe) [41]. Table 3.1 gives examples of estimated CO_2e emissions per person per year for selected nations.

These figures give a clear sense of the relative carbon emission burdens that different nations of the world impose on the atmosphere. Since we as individuals contribute to these figures, how can we get a better sense of the carbon costs of our personal activities? Attempts to do this are confounded by the earlier observation of systems and their 'hidden parts'; carbon dioxide is invisible, and it is generally hard to get a sense of the weight of a gas. Hence, it may help to compare our individual annual carbon 'output' to other better known objects. For instance, a small car weighs around 1000 kg, so in the United Kingdom citizens create on average, per person, the weight of fifteen cars of carbon dioxide per annum. To find out more about the carbon footprints of individual acts or products we recommend the book *How Bad are Bananas?* by Mike Berners-Lee; Table 3.2 gives some examples [42].

Consider that a pint of petrol, when burned, creates approximately 1 kg of carbon dioxide. Is it not extraordinary, then, to think that having a bath requires the combustion of two and a half pints of petrol? Running a bath, eating a burger and drinking a bottle of water a day would move us close to our personal allowance of two tonnes per year for sustainable usage. With these sobering sums in mind, many of the coming chapters are concerned

Table 3.2 Estimated average carbon footprints of selected products or activities [42].

Product or activity	CO$_2$e
A pint of tap water	0.14 g
500 ml of bottled water	215 g (travelling 600 miles by road)
A large bath using water heated by electricity	2.6 kg
A 4-ounce cheeseburger	2.5 kg
Flying to from London to Glasgow and back	500 kg
Heart bypass operation	1100 kg
A person	From 0.1 tonne (average Malawian) to 30 tonnes (average Australian) per year
Having a child	From 100 tonnes (a carbon conscious child) to 373 tonnes (average) to 2000 tonnes (high-impact offspring) over their lifetime
A university	72 000 tonnes per year
The Football World Cup	2.8 million tonnes (South Africa World Cup)
The world's data centres	130 million tonnes (2010), predicted to rise to 250–340 million tonnes for 2020

with ways of managing and reducing the carbon footprint of healthcare through personal, practice and policy interventions.

Concluding thoughts

This chapter has attempted to offer a broad and nuanced definition of sustainability. The aim of becoming more sustainable is simple: to improve the current state of the planet and leave it in a fit state for future generations. The *process* of sustainability is more complex. Sustainability is what happens when systems work well, when we appreciate sources, sinks and cycles, rather than forgetting our open relationship with the Earth system. Understanding systems theory helps us appreciate when a system is healthy and communicating freely within itself and with the systems around it. The same awareness helps us recognise systems that are dysfunctional or *precarious* – seemingly healthy but in fact about to crash. From a healthcare perspective, a key systems concept is that of resilience, the interior capacity of a system (or person) to get well, stay well and adapt to illness when it comes knocking. All healthcare systems should build resilience.

Despite their salience, the ideas of sustainability are slow to catch on. Even with massive progress in this area and notwithstanding the growing number of enthusiastic and committed individuals and organisations, it seems fair to say that we are still awaiting the emergence of a critical mass of active advocates. Even well-informed people who are aware of the negative effects that carbon emissions have on the climate continue with carbon lifestyles far in access of 2000 kg carbon dioxide per annum, and the metaphor of addiction accurately describes this paradox. There is no quick fix but a positive message is more likely to win hearts and minds than a message that reminds us what we cannot do. Healthcare is 'lucky' here, because nearly everything that helps create a healthier planet has the co-benefit of making people healthier and happier. With a clearer sense of sustainability in mind, the following chapters aim to offer a positive vision for sustainable healthcare.

References

1. Brundtland Commission – Wikipedia [Internet]. http://en.wikipedia.org/wiki/Brundtland_Commission [accessed 24 September 2011].
2. Bundy, A.F.P. (2005) Can Atlantic cod (Gadus morhua) recover? Exploring trophic explanations for the non-recovery of the cod stock on the eastern Scotian Shelf, Canada. *Canadian Journal of Fisheries and Aquatic Sciences*, **62**, 1474–1489.
3. Meadows, D.H. and Wright, D. (2009) *Thinking in Systems: A Primer.* Earthscan Ltd, London.
4. Winchester, S. (1998) *The River at the Centre of the World: A Journey Up the Yangtze, and Back in Chinese Time.* Penguin Books Ltd.
5. Greenblatt, M., Becerra, R.M. and Serafetinides, E.A. (1982) Social networks and mental health: on overview. *American Journal of Psychiatry*, **139** (8), 977–984.
6. Berkman, L.F. and Syme, S.L (1979) Social networks, host resistance, and mortality: a nine-year follow-up study of Alameda County residents. *American Journal of Epidemiology*, **109** (2), 186–204.
7. Bilchick, K.C., Fetics, B., Djoukeng, R. *et al.* (2002) Prognostic value of heart rate variability in chronic congestive heart failure (Veterans Affairs' Survival Trial of Antiarrhythmic Therapy in Congestive Heart Failure). *American Journal of Cardiology*, **90** (1), 24–28.
8. Marais, E.N. (2009) *The Soul of the White Ant.* New York University Press.
9. Kauffman, S.A. (1996) *At Home in the Universe: The Search for Laws of Self-organisation and Complexity.* Penguin Books Ltd.
10. Lovelock, J. (2000) *Gaia: A New Look at Life on Earth.* Oxford Paperbacks.
11. Lovelock, J.E. and Margulis, L (1974) Atmospheric homeostasis by and for the biosphere: the gaia hypothesis. *Tellus*, **26** (1–2), 2–10.
12. Midgley, M. (2007) *Earthy Realism: The Meaning of Gaia.* Imprint Academic.
13. Lovelock, J. (2009) *The Vanishing Face of Gaia: a Final Warning.* Viking Adult.
14. Huber, M., Knottnerus, J.A., Green L *et al.* (2011) How should we define health? *British Medical Journal*, **343**, d4163.

15. Thompson, T. (2011) Resilience - a concept comes of age. *Journal of Holistic Healthcare*, **8** (2), 19–22.
16. Oxford English Dictionary – resilience, n. [Internet]. http://www.oed.com/viewdictionaryentry/Entry/163619 [accessed 17 July 2011].
17. Masten, A.S., Best, K.M. and Garmezy, N. (1990) Resilience and Development: Contributions from the Study of Children Who Overcome Adversity. *Development and Psychopathology*, **2** (04), 425–444.
18. Holling, C.S., Carpenter, S.R., Kinzig, A. and Walker, B. (2004) Resilience, Adaptability and Transformability in Social-Ecological Systems. *Ecology and Society*, **9** (2), 5.
19. Putnam, R. (2001) *Bowling Alone: The Collapse and Revival of American Community*. Simon & Schuster Ltd.
20. Norberg, J. and Cumming, G.S. (2008) *Complexity theory for a sustainable future*. Columbia University Press.
21. Smith, R., Gross, K. and Robertson, G. (2008) Effects of Crop Diversity on Agroecosystem Function: Crop Yield Response. *Ecosystems*, **11** (3), 355–366.
22. Raffle, A.E. (2010) Oil, health, and health care. *British Medical Journal*, **341**, c4596–c4596.
23. Eriksson, M. (2011) Social capital and health – implications for health promotion. *Global Health Action*, **4**, 5611.
24. The World Bank (2009) Public attitudes toward climate change: findings from a multi-country poll. World Development Report 2010. *The World Bank*, Washington, DC.
25. GALLUP (2010) 'Jobs' Drops to No. 2 on Americans' List of Top Problems [Internet]. http://www.gallup.com/poll/127949/jobs-drops-no-americans-list-top-problems.aspx [accessed 19 September 2011].
26. Mayfield, D., McLeod, G. and Hall, P. (1974) The CAGE questionnaire: validation of a new alcoholism screening instrument. *American Journal of Psychiatry*, **131** (10), 1121–1123.
27. Prochaska, J.O. and DiClemente, C.C. (1986) Toward a comprehensive model of change. In: W.R. Miller, and N. Heather, (eds.) *Treating addictive behaviors: processes of change*, pp. 3–27. Plenum Press, New York.
28. Kubler-Ross, E. and Kessler D. (2005) On Grief and Grieving: *Finding the Meaning of Grief Through the Five Stages of Loss*. Simon & Schuster Ltd.
29. Johnstone, C. (2011) Understanding denial. Can insights from the addictions treatments help us tackle ecological crisis? *Journal of Holistic Health*, **8** (2), 27–30.
30. Macy, J. and Johnstone, C. (2012) *Active Hope: How to Face the Mess We're in without Going Crazy*. New World Library, Novato, CA.
31. Maller, C., Townsend, M., Pryor, A., Brown, P. and St, Leger L. (2006) Healthy nature healthy people: 'contact with nature' as an upstream health promotion intervention for populations. *Health Promotion International*, **21** (1), 45–54.
32. Bacon, F. (2008) *Francis Bacon: The Major Works*. OUP, Oxford.
33. Chatwin, B. (2008) *The Songlines*. Vintage Classics.
34. der Post L.V. (1964) The Lost World of the Kalahari. Penguin Books Ltd.
35. Page, J. (2004) *In the Hands of the Great Spirit: The 20, 000 Year History of American Indians*. Simon & Schuster Ltd.

36. Kaptchuk, T.J. (2000) *Chinese Medicine: The Web That Has No Weaver*, 2nd revised edn. Contemporary (McGraw-Hill), Chicago, IL.

37. Astley, N. (2007) *Earth Shattering: ecopoems*. Bloodaxe Books Ltd.

38. Ganten, D., Haines, A. and Souhami, R. (2010) Health co-benefits of policies to tackle climate change. *Lancet*, **376** (9755), 1802–1804.

39. CO_2 Now (Home) [Internet]. http://co2now.org/ [accessed 21 September 2011].

40. Padgett, J.P., Steinemann, A.C., Clarke, J.H. and Vandenbergh, M.P. (2008) A comparison of carbon calculators. *Environmental Impact Assessment Review*, **28** (2–3), 106–115.

41. Hertwich, E.G. and Peters, G.P. (2009) Carbon Footprint of Nations: A Global, Trade-Linked Analysis. *Environmental Science & Technology*, **43** (16), 6414–6420.

42. Berners-Lee, M. (2010) *How Bad Are Bananas?: The carbon footprint of everything*. Profile Books, London.

Chapter 4 **A vision for sustainable healthcare**

In this chapter

- Redefining value and health
- Why should health services become more sustainable?
- What will sustainable healthcare look and feel like?

Redefining *value* and *health* in healthcare

The ecological impact of healthcare delivery is only one part of the vision of a truly holistic and sustainable system of prevention, cure and care. Creating more sustainable health systems also involves reconsidering and redefining what *value* means to us. Entities promoted as being 'valuable' are often those that carry a high price; for example, stylish clothes, luxury cars and long-haul flights. As well as being expensive, these things incur high carbon costs, produce waste and deplete resources. In contrast, sustainable healthcare emphasises different values, many of which are virtually limitless, such as compassion, kindness, being caring, having fun, maintaining friendships, holding conversations, viewing nature or being mindful. All of these also have clear health benefits.

The nature, prevalence and meaning of health and disease have changed in recent years, and so has the context for sustainable development (which we define later in this chapter). Health services now increasingly deal with multisystem risk factors for chronic diseases that define the 'modern world', and some previous concepts of 'ill' and 'well' have now largely become outmoded. Not surprisingly, the question of 'What is health?' continues to be the subject of debate. Jadad and colleagues, writing in the *British Medical Journal* in 2011, proposed a new definition of health as being 'the ability to adapt and self-manage' in the face of social, physical and emotional

Sustainable Healthcare, First Edition. Knut Schroeder, Trevor Thompson, Kathleen Frith and David Pencheon.
© 2013 John Wiley & Sons, Ltd. Published 2013 by John Wiley & Sons, Ltd.

challenges [1]. The same is relevant to other areas: organisations that survive and prosper in the future are not necessarily those which are the biggest or most prestigious – they are, in fact, the ones that deliver today and at the same time adapt for tomorrow. Accordingly, defining what health means is important if health services want to become more sustainable. This requires us to take a fresh look in this and later chapters at what we mean by better health, better end-of-life care and better ways to die.

Why should health services become more sustainable?

Although health systems prevent, cure and manage health problems, they can also *create* health problems in ways we are familiar with (for example, relating to patient safety) and ways with which we are less familiar, such as contributing to climate change. The World Health Organization's Director of Public Health and Environment, Maria Neira, highlighted this paradox when she wrote in *Healthy Hospitals, Healthy Planet, Healthy People*: 'Hospitals are energy and resource intensive enterprises that, as they operate today, contribute substantially to climate change while inadvertently contributing to respiratory and other illnesses' [2]. In this document, the *World Health Organization* and *Health Care Without Harm* also clearly outline the important role that health services play in *mitigating* climate change (that is, reducing the magnitude and consequences of climate change).

Hospitals and community-based healthcare providers need considerable amounts of energy and resources to provide clinical care and operate smoothly. Supplying medicines, procuring food and other goods for patient care and using resources like natural gas for heating and petrol for transporting patients also carries a substantial carbon footprint (Box 4.1).

The figures on energy use in the health sector (even if they may be difficult to comprehend) illustrate that the healthcare community uses up substantial resources [2]. As a result, health systems directly and indirectly cause some of the illnesses and health problems that they try to prevent and treat, so clearly contradict one of the main guiding ethical principles in healthcare, *primum non nocere – first do no harm* (or at least ensure that the short and long-term benefits far outweigh the short and long-term harms). Energy consumption is only part of health services' carbon footprint, because it does not take into consideration the carbon emissions that the health sector incurs through, for example, use of medical equipment, information technology, food and medication. Although calculating the *exact* carbon footprint of any health service around the world is impossible, the estimates unequivocally suggest that it is very large indeed. This leaves no doubt that by reducing carbon emissions and making better use of resources, health systems can not

Box 4.1   Health systems and carbon emissions: example statistics

- In 2007, the US health care sector accounted for 16% of US gross domestic product and was responsible for 8% of total US greenhouse gas emissions [3].
- In the United Kingdom, the National Health Service (NHS) calculated that its annual carbon emissions in 2007 were more than 21 million tonnes of CO_2e, which is about a quarter of all emissions from the public sector in the United Kingdom [4]. Broken down, procurement topped the list of individual contributions with 60%, followed by building energy (22%) and travel (18%).
- According to the US Department of Energy, US hospitals use 836 trillion British Thermal Units (BTUs) of energy at a cost of US$ 5 billion (£3.2 billion) every year, which is more than double the energy use and carbon emissions of all standard US office buildings [3].
- In Brazil, hospitals consume an estimated 10% of the total commercial energy [5].

only contribute to mitigating climate change, they will also help improve population health while doing so. So addressing the ecological impact of healthcare delivery is an important part of the vision for a truly holistic and sustainable healthcare system achieving prevention, cure and care.

Addressing inefficiencies in health provision

Inefficiencies are common in the health sector, even in technologically and economically advanced countries. For instance, the US health system, though in many respects forward-thinking and competitive, has been described as inefficient not only because of its high administrative costs and the fragmented care it sometimes provides, but also because of the differences in the quality of treatment for patients, depending on race, income and where they live [6]. Because there is no 'perfect' health service and inefficiencies are widely prevalent, there is always room for making improvements. Using resources responsibly and working more effectively are, therefore, important components of sustainable healthcare, which not only help the health sector reduce its carbon footprint but also make financial savings, improve compliance with legislation, increase resilience and, most importantly, improve quality of care.

Responding to national frameworks, targets and international initiatives

Another reason for health services to get their own house in order when it comes to tackling climate change is the legally mandated target to reduce national carbon emissions. Organisations in the United Kingdom, for example, need to demonstrate that their governance arrangements conform with government targets to reduce emissions by 80% by 2050 compared to levels in 1990 [7]. The United States has committed to reducing its greenhouse gas emissions to 17% below 2005 levels by 2020 [8]. And the European Commission aims to reduce greenhouse gas emissions by 8% below 1990 levels by 2008–2012 [9] (Box 4.2). Similar regulations apply also in many other countries. Consequently, healthcare institutions as well as other public bodies come under increasing scrutiny to demonstrate their commitment to actions about climate change, which is a good reason for trying to be ahead of the game.

Achieving all-round benefits

The evidence grows that by tackling global environmental problems, health services can improve population health on a wider scale. In 2009, *The Lancet* published a landmark series of papers that illustrates the sometimes striking short-term health benefits that can be gained from actions to tackle climate

---

Box 4.2   Implementing sustainable development at international level

A number of countries have developed strategies to implement sustainable development. The Division of Sustainable Development (DSD) of the UN Department of Economic and Social Affairs provides leadership and expertise at international level within the United Nations on sustainable development [10]. The UK government published its strategy document *Securing the Future* in 2005, promoting a more sustainable economy, the responsible use of sound science, and good governance [11]. The priority areas laid out in this document include sustainable consumption and production, climate change and energy, protecting natural resources and the environment, as well as creating sustainable communities in a fairer world. In the United States, the Bureau of Oceans and International Environmental and Scientific Affairs of the US Department of State lead a number of partnerships and initiatives that promote economic growth, social development and environmental stewardship [12].

change [13–22]. These are, of course, not isolated reports, and many other publications have, before and since, pointed out both the need for the health sector to act, as well as the benefits to be gained from actions against global environmental change.

What is sustainable healthcare?

Achieving sustainable healthcare is a continuous journey, known as *sustainable development* (Chapter 3 also details more on what sustainability means). This journey is about making sure that our actions and decisions include 'development that meets the needs of the present without compromising the ability of future generations to meet their own needs', a definition originally coined in the 1987 *World Commission on Environment and Development Report* (also known as the *Brundtland Commission*), titled *'Our Common Future'* [23]. Sustainable healthcare is a way of providing care that is 'living and working within our means' with regard to natural resources at its core. It is healthcare that avoids putting detrimental stress on environmental and human systems which not only endanger the health of the current global population but also negatively affect the health and wellbeing of generations in the future (and elsewhere now) [24].

To better engage with the concept of sustainable development, it helps to create a visual picture in our minds as to what sustainable healthcare means in practice. The *UK NHS Sustainable Development Unit* outlines a number of distinct positive features and characteristics of a sustainable healthcare system that help to create such a picture (Figure 4.1), in which the notion of 'addressing needs today without prejudicing our ability to do the same in future' is crucial [25].

In a sustainable healthcare system, everyone does their best to provide the best quality of care, promote healthy living and minimise the human impact on the environment. Above all, the scale of the challenge and the scale of the opportunities mean more than just seeking and delivering efficiencies. In fact, we need to constantly re-examine the whole rationale and business case for how we maintain health and address illness.

Components of a more sustainable and holistic health sector

It is impossible to predict exactly what our future and that of health services will look like. Even so, organisations such as the *Forum for the Future* and the *UK National Health Service Sustainable Development Unit* have developed scenarios and predictions that try to illustrate what healthcare in a less carbon dependent and more resource-aware future may be like (Box 4.3 gives some examples) [26].

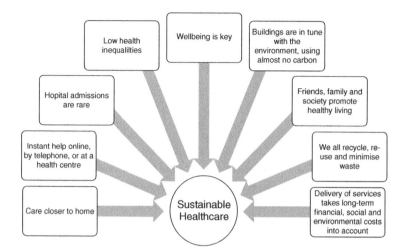

Figure 4.1   Likely features of a sustainable healthcare system. (Data from [26].)

Box 4.3   Possible features of more sustainable societies (adapted from *Fit For the Future*)[26]

- The high price of carbon has created a new type of consumerist world where businesses sell services (for example, wellness coaching) rather than products (such as pharamaceuticals), and good citizens share with their neighbours.
- Communities work together to support healthy lifestyles, and business takes increasing responsibility for promoting public health.
- Countries prioritise economic and social resilience over growth, and quality of life is the key goal.
- People value meaningful work, low-impact lifestyles and their community.
- Healthy living is a high priority, and much care is delivered through friends, families and charities.
- Workplace health schemes are common.
- Rapid innovation and novel technologies have created a low-carbon economy.

We are likely to see 12 themes in some form in a more sustainable and low-carbon health system (Table 4.1) [27].

The following sections give a brief introduction and overview of how some these themes can be integrated into health systems (the later chapters go into more detail).

Models of care

More sustainable healthcare systems are likely to invest and engage much more in preventive care. One important factor for achieving this is a better integration of health services with various other sectors. These may include, for instance, community networks, housing/planning/transport departments and educational organisations, which ideally need to contribute to and be part of a fully integrated health system. Sustainable health systems will only be viable as a part of sustainable communities [28]. Examples would be to provide better and more energy efficient housing for vulnerable people (for instance through fitting roof insulation and draft-proof windows and doors) as part of a combined approach, or working with local authorities to encourage active travel by prioritising investment in cycle paths and public transport to make it easier for people to choose active travel over car use [29]. This would not only contribute to improving people's health but also improve people's lives in the long run by saving energy and money.

In future models of care, people will work smarter, not harder. Although we cannot exactly predict what health services will look like in the future, they are likely to be very different from the traditional services we see today. Reasons for this include both classic drivers of change, such as changing demography, the development of new technologies and different expectations (including clinicians as well as patients and the public), and *new* drivers, such as resource limitation, globalisation, and environmental change (including climate change) [30].

Future hospitals, for example, may become very different places, with more emphasis on health than disease. Hospitals may be also become smaller, more targeted to the needs of the population they serve, and so become more part of the local community. As we will explore in the next chapter, hospital services may even become redundant in some respects, and more care will be provided in the community and in people's homes. Research will play an important role in this process by informing the development of evidence that supports modifying models of care.

Table 4.1 Healthcare themes in a sustainable future. (Data from [28].)

Theme	Features
1 Considering cost, benefit and value	Accounting for the costs, benefits and the genuine value of whole systems – both now and in the future; gaining benefits from acting on root causes rather than 'symptoms'.
2 Connecting healthy people and healthy places	Making the connection between healthy people and healthy places; fostering stronger, diverse and more resilient communities [29].
3 Achieving a different attitude to end of life and death	Creating a culture where death is more 'normal' and people have more control over their final days (see also Chapter 10 on Sustainable Death).
4 Learning across communities and countries	Encouraging learning between richer and poorer countries; moving towards a culturally and spiritually richer life [30].
5 Aligning incentives and maximising co-benefits	Bringing incentives and benefits into line, including financial, personal, professional, economic and social.
6 Addressing social equality	Tackling the wellbeing and opportunities of the least empowered, taking into account what is good for long-term sustainability; using resources equitably.
7 Improving the quality of healthcare	Concentrating on providing high quality healthcare, taking into account the benefits and risks for the future.
8 Preventing illness	Considering avoidable illness as a system failure – and acting upon it.
9 Doing more good than harm	Striving towards a system that avoids harming people, resources and the environment – and that does much more good.
10 Connecting communities	Helping communities to connect with each other and consume less.
11 Understanding efficiency and transformational change	Addressing efficiency (doing the same but with less resource to achieve better outcomes) and transformational change (doing fundamentally different things with less resources to achieve better outcomes, reviewing and if necessary revising of how to achieve core objectives); increasing transparency.

(continued overleaf)

Table 4.1 (*continued*)

Theme	Features
12 Improving communication and empowering people	Using technology to its best effect to improve communication within and between communities so that they feel more empowered; helping people to become more comfortable with the degree of control and autonomy over their own lives and deaths [31].

Sustainability governance in healthcare

Apart from looking different, hospitals and other healthcare settings in the future may also be less hierarchical, with more skill and task sharing by professionals for whom sustainability is as important as high quality of care and financial governance. Healthcare managers and other people working in the health sector will see themselves as members of organisations that take their environmental, social and financial responsibilities seriously. Part of this process will be consistent reporting in all the areas relevant to sustainability through a Board-approved (and regularly reviewed) Sustainable Development Management Plan (SDMP), and being prepared for comparisons against agreed standards and other organisations [31]. The healthcare sector (and healthcare professionals such as doctors and nurses in particular) needs to *lead* by example. Various organisations, such as *Healthcare Without Harm*, the *Climate and Health Council, Swedish Doctors for the Environment* or *Doctors for the Environment Australia*, are examples of initiatives that encourage health professionals to take up the cause for sustainable development and help with this process [32–34].

The co-benefits of sustainability actions

When health services consider sustainability in all their actions, they not only incur environmental benefits, but can also produce significant direct and indirect health, social and economic rewards. Referred to as the *triple bottom line* (easily remembered as '*people, planet, profit*'), these co-benefits from increased sustainability make a compelling case for the health sector to engage in environmentally friendly actions. These three components often work in synergy rather than in isolation, because it is their relationship to the whole that signifies their importance (Figure 4.2) [35].

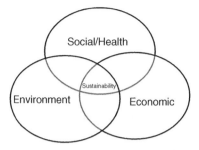

Figure 4.2   Important components of sustainability: the triple bottom line. (Data from [36].)

Tight finances are often seen as a major stumbling block when it comes to plans for making health services more sustainable. Fortunately, reducing the carbon footprint and making better use of resources does not always have to come at a price for healthcare providers but may, on the contrary, create opportunities for potentially substantial savings, as the selected examples in the following sections demonstrate (we present more case studies and examples in the topic-specific later chapters).

Potential gains from energy savings

As prices of fossil fuels will rise in the future, saving energy, using energy more efficiently and optimising the use of alternative energy often makes good environmental as well as financial sense. This is particularly relevant for healthcare providers that already struggle with meeting their energy demands because of limited resources, or in areas where traditional fossil fuels are costly (Box 4.4).

Box 4.4   Example of hospital energy costs in the United States

Estimates from the *Practice Greenhealth Energy Impact Calculator (EIC)* indicate that a typical 200-bed hospital in coal-powered areas in the US Midwest uses about seven million kWh per year. Consequently, such a hospital is responsible for over US$ 1 million (£629 000) per year in negative societal public health impacts, and US$ 107 000 (£67 000) per year in direct healthcare costs [36]. Although such figures can only be estimates, there is little doubt that positive health impacts are likely to be substantial where health services manage to improve their energy efficiency and change to more environmentally friendly sources of energy.

> **Case study 4.1　Optimised energy management in India**
>
> One of the largest and oldest hospitals in South-East Asia, the Sir Jamshedji Jeejeebhoy (Sir J.J.) Hospital in Mumbai, India, achieved a reduction in energy costs through better energy management. Being a busy and modern hospital that operates 24 hours a day, energy bills – not surprisingly – run high. The hospital's operating theatres, top-end medical equipment, lighting, high-voltage alternating current systems, water heaters, elevators and water pumps contribute to more than 75% of the total energy bill. In 2001, the hospital authorities took action on a prime ministerial call to conserve energy by aiming to raise awareness about inefficient energy use. The campaign, which used posters, slogans and other measures, was a striking success. By systematically switching off office equipment, repairing leaks in the air conditioning and making better use of natural daylight, the hospital saved 812 000 kWh of electricity between 2002 and 2004 [37]. This reduced the hospital's energy bill by an impressive US$ 90 000 (£58 000) – an amount that could pay for around 475 cataract operations in India assuming a cost of about 10 000 Rs (£122 or US$ 188) each, thus freeing up resources for improving patient care and other activities.

Using alternative forms of energy that reduce dependence on fossil fuels is often particularly relevant for large urban hospitals (where changes in fuel prices and supplies can have great consequences because of the amounts of fuel being used) as well as for remote clinics, where these rely on reliable delivery of fuel to function. Many examples exist where using energy more effectively not only saves carbon but also creates financial savings (Case studies 4.1 and 4.2).

Energy bills – and so carbon emissions – can be equally high for healthcare providers in Europe and North America, where making better use of the available energy creates fascinating stories, too.

These case studies are not isolated examples, and many other carbon and energy reducing schemes around the world have shown that substantial amounts of money can be saved, which then can be re-diverted to patient care and other priorities [32].

The benefits of better food management

Health services buy and distribute food in large quantities. When healthcare providers such as hospitals move towards a more plant-based diet for their patients and staff and reduce animal products like meat and dairy

Case study 4.2   Improved energy efficiency in the United Kingdom

For the managers and clinicians at the Renal Unit at the Royal Cornwall Hospital, UK, sustainability actions proved a great success – environmentally, financially and clinically. By identifying ways to improve efficiency and change the way they provide care, they set out to reduce their carbon footprint [38]. The results were staggering. By the end of the first year, they achieved carbon reductions of around 33 tonnes of CO_2e per year – roughly the equivalent to around 66 return flights from London to Madrid. But not only that – at the same time they also improved the patient experience, with about 50% less waiting, reduced journeys and more self-care. The benefits of their actions did not stop here; staff had more time to look after patients, healthcare acquired infections were reduced and the unit achieved cost savings of £1200 (US$ 2000) per employee per year. After two years, additional actions reduced CO_2e emissions by 53 tonnes. Simeon Edwards, Unit Manager, must have been delighted when he reportedly said: 'We now have cost avoidances running at over £57 000 (US$ 91 000) a year as a result of this carbon reduction programme. It would be wonderful if we could re-invest some of that into more carbon reductions'.

in the meals they serve, in the longer term they are likely to contribute to reducing methane levels (an important greenhouse gas) from farming. In addition to being more environmentally friendly, a more plant-based diet has less saturated fat, with obvious direct health benefits. In addition, buying fresh and locally produced seasonal products takes less energy to produce, particularly because of reduction in 'food miles' – and is also good for people's health. Health practitioners also have a great opportunity by advocating a more plant-based diet to their patients. The co-benefits around using food in new and more sustainable ways are often easily accessible and persuasive (there is more on food in Chapter 6).

Co-benefits from active travel

Travel is another area where co-benefits of sustainability actions are easy to identify (there is more on this in Chapter 7). Moving staff and patients is an integral part of providing traditional patient care in most settings. Often this involves carbon-intensive transport, for example in buses or cars. By increasing levels of active travel (such as cycling or walking) in those people who are able to do so, health services can contribute to lowering transport energy-use and reducing carbon emissions and pollution. Active travel helps improve the health of the people who get around this way, because it lowers their risk of heart disease, obesity, diabetes and mild mental illness – and also helps reduce road traffic crashes [39, 40].

Increasing the number of people who cycle is an obvious area for boosting active travel [41]. Cycling is very energy efficient and allows people to travel an about 10-times wider range compared to walking. Cycling is also cheap, as it does not incur any fuel costs, and the maintenance costs for a bicycle are much lower than for cars. Consequently, encouraging health professionals and patients (those who are able to cycle) to travel more actively is a good starting point.

Increasing active and low-carbon travel also makes a compelling case for health services to help improve air quality. A systematic review conducted by the World Health Organization estimates that exposure to fine particle matter in outdoor air leads to about 100 000 deaths and 725 000 years of life lost each year in Europe [42]. Consequently, reducing the environmental impact of carbon-intensive travel in the healthcare sector should be a priority for the healthcare community, particularly in heavily polluted areas (there is more about the positive effects from more sustainable movement of people and goods in Chapter 7).

Monitoring and reducing carbon emissions

At present, measuring sustainable development and carbon emissions in the health sector remains a challenge. One reason for this is that in many areas we still lack well-researched, appropriate, relevant and practical metrics that help us evaluate the different elements contributing to all direct and indirect carbon emissions. Only if we have good and standardised metrics in place can we implement robust review and monitoring systems that help minimise resource use across the healthcare sector. Yet there is progress. For example, the *UK National Health Service Sustainable Development Unit* and *Sustainable Development Commission* have been commissioned to prepare a report on the use of carbon metrics for inclusion in regulatory frameworks [43]. With fitting metrics and carbon review and monitoring procedures in place, healthcare organisations will find it easier to include value and cost related to carbon emissions and resource use in all business decisions (Case study 4.3).

Ideally, healthcare organisations around the world need local, regional, national and international legislative frameworks that require public sustainability reporting as a key responsibility. Being accountable for sustainability and routine life cycle costing should be an integral part of good clinical and

---

Case study 4.3   Measuring carbon emissions

The UK West Midlands Cancer Intelligence Unit demonstrates the importance of measuring carbon emissions. This healthcare organisation has pioneered the use of data from its cancer registry along with a Geographical Information System (GIS) to work out the carbon emissions related to treating breast cancer [44]. Figures from 1999 to 2004 indicated a 214% increase in total car miles travelled, which equates to over 400 tons of carbon emissions from radiotherapy treatment in the West Midlands. Reflecting on patient and visitor mileage, and therefore carbon emissions, is thus a useful tool for helping to design lower carbon pathways.

---

organisational governance. The information needs to be transparent and current, and should inform further actions and planning.

One key element of this process is that every healthcare organisation signs up to a Board-approved sustainable development plan that clearly identifies measurable carbon reduction milestones to be achieved. These milestones should be in line with national and international targets and trajectories (for the United Kingdom, for example, this would mean a reduction in carbon emissions by 10% of the 2007 levels by 2015, as a minimum).

Using technology to its best effect

Making best use of technology is an important part of sustainable development. Health services can play a vital role in helping to develop and implement lower carbon technologies, which ideally includes support with funding and providing testing grounds for demonstration projects [26]. Information and communication technology (ICT), renewable energy and low-carbon ways of transporting people and goods are examples areas where the health sector can be influential in implementing, evaluating and spreading best practice about innovations that not only advance sustainable development but also deliver better quality of care. Working closely together with academic institutions as well as organisations that specialise in innovation (which may include both the public and commercial sector) will be paramount (Chapter 10).

Working in partnership

It is difficult to over-emphasize the need for health services to foster and strengthen links with other partner organisations, such as charities, local

Case study 4.4   Working with the commercial sector

An example where partnership between the health and private sectors can work is the Chesterfield Royal NHS Foundation Trust in the United Kingdom. This health organisation teamed up with a commercial firm and entered into a window replacement and ventilation programme that has cut the Trust's carbon emissions by more than 50 tonnes a year [44].

businesses, universities and local authorities, as part of sustainable development [44]. This not only allows exchange of information and the design of better care pathways but also gives leverage in business planning and negotiating new contracts that contribute to sustainable development. Examples include the purchasing of services and goods, making optimal use of renewable energy sources and aiming to provide better and more sustainable public transport for patients and staff (Case study 4.4). Cultivating relationships with pharmaceutical companies that work in ethical and sustainable ways can be useful, particularly where pharmaceutical companies have moved towards providing services for preventing illness rather drugs to treat it.

Alternative ways of financing healthcare

An important aspect of sustainable development is the way healthcare is financed. Where healthcare is rewarded for activity and healthcare providers follow commercial principles, this often encourages unnecessary investigations or treatment. To stimulate sustainable health, we need to align money towards needs, populations and outcomes and much less to individuals and activity. Where large healthcare providers (such as hospitals) receive population and outcome-related budgets, this can provide powerful incentives to align health, financial and environmental outcomes (the *triple bottom line*). This approach can reduce wastage (of resources and unnecessary and sometimes harmful healthcare), improve health outcomes, contain costs and provide more incentive to strengthen the role of primary care and preventive medicine. Examples of these newer more sustainable business models of healthcare, found in Spain, India and the USA, can also sometimes empower patients to have more control over their care – especially when delivered in settings closer to home (where partnership and information sharing is vital) rather than within the often impersonal and depersonalising atmosphere of a large hospital [2].

Efficiency at the start of sustainable practice

Efficiency measures are a crucial first part of making health services more sustainable. Healthcare organisations that try to improve the quality of care for their patients can do this by becoming more efficient and productive. Increased efficiency has crucial sustainability implications, so making significant and lasting efficiency changes when transforming healthcare systems not only benefits patients but also individual organisations and the wider healthcare community.

Improvements tend to be easier to implement and are longer-lasting if they are driven by staff themselves. So it is important to help staff with asking difficult questions about their own practice and empowering them to make positive changes to the way they work. A continuous improvement culture can lead to real savings in materials, reducing waste and improving staff morale. The *NHS Institute for Innovation and Improvement*, for example, has pioneered methods and techniques for achieving this in secondary care settings and also in primary care and community centres, many of which have been adapted from models used in industry (such as 'lean' technology) [45]. Efficiency is vital and is often a good entry point or introduction to making health systems more sustainable. Efficiency gives organisations, leaders and staff the confidence and skills to progress to more transformational changes in the way health care is organised.

Although sustainable development often creates valuable co-benefits along the triple bottom line, this is of course not always the case. In reality, making healthcare more sustainable may sometimes require changes that we may not immediately perceive as appealing, particularly in areas where we have got used to a certain way of living and working (air travel is an obvious example). But sustainable development is a necessary response to the 'stresses' that we (as health services and as the global community) face. We now have the option to collaborate in inspiring way to tackle these challenges, difficult as it occasionally may be – or we face the prospect of fierce or even violent competition further down the line.

The first three chapters of this book set out to define the ecological crises that healthcare faces in the coming decades and the principles of sustainability that might help us mitigate and adapt to the problems that lie ahead. In this chapter we have taken these principles and woven them into a vision for sustainable healthcare. This vision may at first glance seem utopian but, as the examples in this chapter (which are only a small selection) have shown, many successful initiatives have been implemented or are under way that provide healthcare in more sustainable and much better ways. But much more needs to be done so that we *will* have a truly lower-carbon healthcare system in thirty years from now. To achieve this, all of us working in or with the healthcare sector need to wake up to this challenge and engage with this transition towards a sustainable healthcare system. Ideally, this process of transition will be measured and active rather than traumatic and unexpected. And because sustainability issues are so closely linked to health, it seems right that the healthcare sector should take a lead and show a good example to the rest of society. The remainder of this book is about unpacking this vision and giving ideas of best practice in areas such as transport, healthy eating, end-of-life care and resource management. Finally, we will discuss ways of bringing the sustainability vision into healthcare education and look at ways of how we can implement this vision on a larger scale. But we begin with what will be most relevant for clinicians: low-carbon clinical care.

Key points

- Healthcare is part of the problem as well as the solution with regard to global environmental change.
- Plenty of reasons exist why the healthcare community needs to engage in sustainability, including legally binding frameworks, co-benefits and current inefficiencies.
- Health professions should lead by example.
- Key to sustainable healthcare is to make healthcare more efficient.
- Sustainable healthcare is low-carbon, supports self-care, makes better use of information and communication technology, and focuses on illness prevention rather than treatment.

References

1. Huber, M., Knottnerus, J.A., Green, L. *et al.* (2011) How should we define health? *British Medical Journal*, 343, d4163.
2. World Health Organization and Healthcare Without Harm (2009) Healthy hospitals, healthy planet, healthy people: Addressing climate change in healthcare settings [Internet]. http://www.who.int/globalchange/publications/climatefoot print_report.pdf [accessed 30 July 2011].
3. US Department of Energy (2009) Department of Energy Announces the Launch of the Hospital Energy Alliance to Increase Energy Efficiency in the Healthcare Sector [Internet]. http://www.doe.gov/articles/department-energy-announces-launch-hospital-energy-alliance-increase-energy-efficiency [accessed 30 July 2011].
4. NHS (2008) NHS England Carbon Emissions Carbon Footprinting Report [Internet]. http://www.sd-commission.org.uk/data/files/publications/NHS_Carbon_ Emissions_modelling1.pdf [accessed 30 July 2011].

5. Szklo, A. (2004) Energy consumption indicators and CHP technical potential in the Brazilian hospital sector. *Energy Conversion and Management*, **45** (13–14), 2075–2091.
6. Garber, A.M. and Skinner, J. (2008) Is American Health Care Uniquely Inefficient? *Journal of Economic Perspectives*, **22** (4), 27–50.
7. Climate Change Act 2008 [Internet]. http://www.legislation.gov.uk/ukpga/2008/27/part/1 [accessed 30 July 2011].
8. World Resources Institute – U.S. Climate Action [Internet]. http://www.wri.org/project/us-climate-action [accessed 30 July 2011].
9. European Commission – Climate Action: Greenhouse gas monitoring and reporting [Internet].http://ec.europa.eu/clima/policies/g-gas/index_en.htm [accessed 30 July 2011].
10. UN Department of Economic and Social Affairs – Division For Sustainable Development: About [Internet]. http://www.un.org/esa/dsd/dsd/dsd_index.shtml [accessed 31 July 2011].
11. UK Government (2005) Securing the future: delivering UK sustainable development strategy [Internet].http://www.defra.gov.uk/publications/files/pb10589-securing-the-future-050307.pdf [accessed 31 July 2011].
12. US Department of State – Sustainable Development [Internet]. http://www.state.gov/e/oes/sus/ [accessed 31 July 2011].
13. Horton, R. (2009)The climate dividend. *Lancet*, **374** (9705), 1869–1870.
14. Chan, M. (2009) Cutting carbon, improving health. *Lancet*, **374** (9705), 1870–1871.
15. Gill, M. and Stott, R. (2009) Health professionals must act to tackle climate change. *Lancet*, **374** (9706), 1953–1955.
16. Haines, A., Wilkinson, P., Tonne, C. and Roberts, I. (2010)Aligning climate change and public health policies. *Lancet*, **374** (9707), 2035–2038.
17. Wilkinson, P., Smith, K.R., Davies, M. *et al.* (2009) Public health benefits of strategies to reduce greenhouse-gas emissions: household energy. *Lancet*, 2009 **374** (9705), 1917–1929.
18. Woodcock, J., Edwards, P., Tonne, C. *et al.* (2009) Public health benefits of strategies to reduce greenhouse-gas emissions: urban land transport. *Lancet*, **374** (9705), 1930–1943.
19. Markandya, A., Armstrong, B.G., Hales, S. *et al.* (2009) Public health benefits of strategies to reduce greenhouse-gas emissions: low-carbon electricity generation. *Lancet*, **374** (9706), 2006–2015.
20. Friel, S., Dangour, A.D., Garnett, T. *et al.* (2009) Public health benefits of strategies to reduce greenhouse-gas emissions: food and agriculture. *Lancet*, **374** (9706), 2016–2025.
21. Smith, K.R., Jerrett, M., Anderson, H.R. *et al.* (2010) Public health benefits of strategies to reduce greenhouse-gas emissions: health implications of short-lived greenhouse pollutants. *Lancet.* **374** (9707), 2091–2103.
22. Haines, A., McMichael, A.J., Smith, K.R. *et al.* (2010) Public health benefits of strategies to reduce greenhouse-gas emissions: overview and implications for policy makers. *Lancet*, **374** (9707), 2104–2114.

23. World Commission on Environment and Development (1987) *Our common future*. Oxford University Press, Oxford.
24. UK Faculty of Public Health (2009) Sustaining a healthy future: taking action on climate change. UK Faculty of Public Health, London.
25. NHS Sustainable Development Unit (2011) Route Map for Sustainable Health. NHS Sustainable Development Unit, Cambridge.
26. NHS Sustainable Development Unit (2009) Fit for the Future [Internet]. http://www.sdu.nhs.uk/publications-resources/4/Fit-for-the-Future-/ [accessed 6 August 2011].
27. Pencheon, D. (2011) Towards a lower carbon health system. *Journal of Holistic Healthcare*, **8** (2), 15–18.
28. Warburton, D. (2009) *Community and Sustainable Development: 6*. Earthscan Ltd, London.
29. Bull, F. and Milton, K. (2011) *Let's Get Moving: a systematic pathway for the promotion of physical activity in a primary care setting* (Let's Get Moving was developed based on National Guidance on effective interventions on physical activity released in the United Kingdom in 2006). *Global Health Promotion*, 18 (1), 59–61.
30. Crisp, N. (2010)*Turning the World Upside Down: The Search for Global Health in the 21st Century*. RSM Press Books, London.
31. NHS Sustainable Development Unit – Sustainable Development Management Plans (SDMP) [Internet]. http://www.sdu.nhs.uk/sd_and_the_nhs/sd-governance/sdmp.aspx [accessed 25 November 2011].
32. Health Care Without Harm (Home) [Internet]. http://www.noharm.org/ [accessed 5 August 2011].
33. Climate Health Council (Home) [Internet]. http://www.climateandhealth.org/ [accessed 3 August 2011].
34. Doctors for the Environment, Australia (Home) [Internet].http://dea.org.au/ [accessed 9 October 2011].
35. Barbier, E.B. (2009) The Concept of Sustainable Economic Development. *Environmental Conservation*, **14**, 101.
36. Healthcare Energy Impact Calculator [Internet]. http://www.eichealth.org/ [accessed 1 August 2011].
37. Energy Conservation Awareness Drive at Sir J. J. Hospital Mumbai, India [Internet]. http://www.pepsonline.org/publications/JJ%20Hospital%20Case%20Study.pdf [accessed 30 July 2011].
38. Centre for Sustainable Healthcare (SAP: Sustainable Action Planning) – Renal Unit, Royal Cornwall Hospital [Internet]. http://sap.greenerhealthcare.org/royal-cornwall-hospital-renal-unit [accessed 26 July 2011].
39. de Nazelle, A., Nieuwenhuijsen, M.J., Antó, J.M. *et al.* (2011) Improving health through policies that promote active travel: a review of evidence to support integrated health impact assessment. *Enviromentn International*, **37** (4), 766–777.
40. WHO (2004) World report on road traffic injury prevention [Internet]. http://www.who.int/violence_injury_prevention/publications/road_traffic/world_report/en/index.html [accessed 23 October 2011].

41. Oja, P., Titze, S., Bauman, A. *et al.* (2011) Health benefits of cycling: a systematic review. *Scandinavian Journal of Medicine & Science in Sports*, **21**, 496–509.

42. European Commission – Clean Air For Europe (café) Reference Documents [Internet].http://ec.europa.eu/environment/archives/cafe/general/keydocs.htm [accessed 1 August 2011].

43. NHS Sustainable Development Unit – NHS Carbon Reduction Strategy: Extended chapters [Internet]. http://www.sdu.nhs.uk/publications-resources/46/NHS-Car bon-Reduction-Strategy--Extended-chapters/ [accessed 18 August 2011].

44. NHS Sustainable Development Unit (2009) Saving Carbon, Improving Health: Carbon Reduction Strategy for England. NHS Sustainable Development Unit, Cambridge.

45. NHS Institute for Innovation and Improvement – The Productive Series [Internet]. http://www.institute.nhs.uk/quality_and_value/productivity_series/the_pro ductive_series.html [accessed 3 August 2011].

Chapter 5 **Low-carbon clinical care**

In this chapter

- Why more sustainable care is better care
- How we can make clinical care more sustainable
- Involving patients
- Better prescribing
- Looking at value in healthcare

More sustainable care is better care

Health professionals around the world work hard to provide effective clinical care. To achieve this, they manage acute illness, deal with chronic conditions, prevent disease and promote better health, which are activities they have been trained to do. But now they also have a new role. Because of the crises faced by health systems all over the world (Chapter 1), responding to the threat of climate change and using resources more effectively is set to become a crucial part of the job.

But it can be difficult to see sustainability as a priority when managing patients does not leave much time and energy for anything else. However, there are good reasons for making clinical care more sustainable in any setting, simply because this will lead to *better* clinical care – care that can lead to substantial clinical, financial and environmental benefits.

Up to now, we have rarely taken into account the substantial environmental costs of delivering care in the way we do [1]. However, current estimates suggest that the benefits of strong, early action on climate change outweigh the fiscal costs; moving to different models of clinical care can play an important role in this process [2]. Sustainability is being increasingly recognised as one of the key dimensions of quality alongside effectiveness, acceptability, efficiency, access, equity and relevance (for instance by the UK Royal College of Physicians) [3]. Sustainability takes a special place among these quality indicators, because it reinforces all of these rather than competing with them

Sustainable Healthcare, First Edition. Knut Schroeder, Trevor Thompson, Kathleen Frith and David Pencheon.
© 2013 John Wiley & Sons, Ltd. Published 2013 by John Wiley & Sons, Ltd.

(a commonly encountered myth that we try to dispel in this and other chapters) [4]. For example, using telephone consultations where appropriate has been shown to be effective in many settings: it reduces travel-related emissions, saves time for patients and practitioners, can improve access to care and is positively valued by patients (for example people with heart failure or HIV) [5, 6].

Health systems also need to become resilient (Chapter 3 gives a full exploration of this term). Being able to manage current and future risks (Chapter 1) effectively is essential for health systems to survive and maintain the capability of providing effective care [7]. This is particularly relevant in settings not only where finances are tight and services suffer energy, fuel and other resource shortages, but also where patient demand is high and human resources in terms of time and skill mix are lacking. Sustainable models of care can help with the transition towards increased resilience.

In this chapter we hope to demonstrate that we *can* deliver clinical care that meets the need of people today in a way that does not compromise the needs of others in the future – and we give some examples of how this can work in practice.

Key areas for making clinical care more sustainable

Even advanced health systems do not always work efficiently [8]. For example, tests are performed or repeated unnecessarily; patients take drugs that they do not need, or receive drugs they do not take; and various health professionals often look after patients' different, but frequently related, medical problems in a disjointed way. The reasons for this ineffective use of resources, such as the desire to benefit an individual, avoid litigation or apply advanced technology to repair bodies, are understandable, but they also mean that health promotion and preventative medicine are often given less importance. Patients also often receive healthcare passively rather than being active participants. As a result, much effort goes into healthcare that is not necessarily related to better outcomes, such as patient satisfaction, quality of life, morbidity or mortality [9].

A number of areas exist where changes in practice would not only lead to better clinical care, but also to overall financial savings and environmental benefits. For example [10, 11]:

- Making effective contraception globally more widely and easily available, thereby reducing the financial, social and environmental effects of unwanted pregnancies.

- More effective prescribing.
- Preventing disease and promoting better health and, thereby, helping people to have fulfilled lives that are meaningful to them whilst living with long-term conditions.
- Educating and empowering patients to allow appropriate self-care and shared decision making with health professionals.
- Re-thinking end-of-life care.
- Making service delivery more efficient and effective ('leaner').
- Using treatments and technologies with lower environmental impact.

Working according to these principles often makes good sense, both clinically and financially, while increasing sustainability. But considering and implementing elements of sustainable clinical care means that we need to be open to changing or even abandoning more traditional ways of practicing medicine.

Providing effective contraception

As discussed in Chapter 1, the global population is growing at an unprecedented rate, putting increasing pressures on the earth's resources and health systems (the estimated average lifetime footprint of a child is around 373 tons of CO_2e, but may be as high as 2000 tons for a high-impact offspring) [12]. Providing effective contraception and educating people about available options to prevent unwanted pregnancies in particular are, therefore, among the biggest contributions the health sector can make to reduce carbon emissions (Chapter 1) and reduce poverty [13]. This is an area where richer countries can provide much support to countries with lower financial resources. According to the UN Population Fund (UNFPA), an estimated 215 million women around the globe (mostly living in the rural areas of sub-Saharan Africa and parts of Southeast Asia, but also in developed countries) want help and support with family planning but are not getting what they need [14]. Consequently, the UNFPA currently focuses on improving reproductive health, empowering women and implementing population and development strategies [15]. At the centre of these activities lies the principle that women have the opportunity to make free and informed decisions about contraception and childbearing (the number, spacing and timing of children). Data from 26 countries show that more highly educated women consistently have lower fertility rates [16]. The UNFPA supports family planning services that [17]:

- Offer a wide selection of methods.
- Reflect high standards of medical practice.
- Are sensitive to cultural conditions.
- Provide sufficient information about proper use and possible side effects.
- Address women's other reproductive health needs.

The ethics of sustainability and individual autonomy may come into conflict when it comes to the number of children people should have. National laws as well as international human rights documents recognise that reproductive rights are human rights, in that couples and individuals should be able to decide freely how many children they want to have and when – and have the right information and resources to do so [18]. While the above strategies help to increase the number of individuals who would like to space or limit their families, they are, of course, not prescriptive about family size. However, it is crucial that people inhabiting this planet are aware that having a child is likely to be the biggest carbon choice they will ever make [12].

Preventing disease and promoting better health

Too often, medicine focuses on diagnosis and treatment, neglecting disease prevention and failing to tackle the social, economic and environmental determinants of ill health [11, 19]. Often we find ourselves fire-fighting, tackling blazes fuelled by our failure to prevent and promote health further back in the causal pathway, while making it unnecessarily difficult for people to help themselves.

Cardiovascular disease, obesity and cancer are examples of big public health problems in many countries all over the world which are, to a large extent, preventable. While these conditions are particularly prevalent in high-income countries, countries that are in transition from being low income to higher income are catching up as populations change their lifestyles towards overeating and under-activity. In addition, vector-borne diseases, such as malaria and gastroenteritis, cause massive disease burdens in lower-income countries – but are also highly preventable.

The evidence base for the effectiveness of interventions that prevent illness is growing constantly. Many good examples can be found in the *Database of Promoting Health Effectiveness Reviews* [DoPHER] [20], which currently hosts details of over 2500 reviews of health promotion and public health effectiveness. Scaling-up water and sanitation services and providing point-of-use disinfection in view of declining global freshwater resources, for instance, are some of these interventions where simple measures can make a tremendous difference to people's lives (Case study 5.1) [21, 22].

> **Case study 5.1   Disease prevention through water sanitation (Data from [21])**
>
> A study conducted by the World Health Organization (WHO) in 2007 found that increasing access to improved water supply and sanitation facilities, increasing access to house-piped water and sewerage connections, and providing household water treatment in ten WHO subregions were cost-effective interventions, especially in developing countries with high mortality rates. Access to piped water supply and sewage connections on plot achieved the highest health impacts, whereas household water treatment was the most cost-effective intervention.

Although not directly measured, interventions like those in Case study 5.1 can often be directly translated into sustainability gains, largely because they help people to lead healthier lives, which reduces the need for curative healthcare.

The effects of clinical decision making

Most clinical decisions (unless they result in a 'wait-and-see' outcome) produce a carbon footprint. Prescribing a drug, ordering an X-ray, referring a patient to a specialist or arranging surgery all have implications in terms of travel and healthcare resource use. It follows that reducing such activities almost invariably helps to reduce carbon emissions and save resources, particularly when actions are unnecessary or of doubtful clinical benefit. An example would be a patient presenting with symptoms suggestive of an uncomplicated upper respiratory infection in primary care. In the majority of cases, this will be due to a simple viral infection, such as the common cold. This common condition is usually self-limiting and does not need further investigation or drug treatment, apart from perhaps symptomatic relief with non-prescription drugs. Yet antibiotic prescribing and ordering of unnecessary investigations like blood tests or X-rays is still widespread, often because of unjustified safety concerns or fear of litigation [23]. Consequently, making evidence-based and appropriate clinical decisions not only helps to avoid costly interventions and treatment but also increases sustainability, particularly where pharmaceuticals are involved.

Rational and responsible prescribing

Prescribing medication is a big part of clinical care and has substantial sustainability implications. Every pill has a life-cycle, from sourcing the ingredients, manufacturing, transport and the disposal of unused medicines. Commonly used ingredients include synthetic petroleum-derived chemicals as well as plant and including animal extracts. Not surprisingly, pharmaceuticals have the biggest impact on the carbon footprint and resource use of health systems. For example, they comprise a fifth of the carbon emissions in the NHS in England [24].

Prescribing medicines inappropriately or unnecessarily and the practice of polypharmacy (especially when patients take more drugs than they need) are widespread and can carry a substantial carbon burden [25]. For example, a report from 2009 concluded that about 145 000 people with dementia in the United Kingdom are wrongly being prescribed antipsychotic medication, which causes an estimated 1800 excess deaths per year [26]. Better prescribing of drugs is, therefore, an area where we can directly and immediately impact on resource use [27]. By choosing treatments that have a more positive environmental and health impact (for example exercise in the treatment of mild to moderate depression), clinical decisions about prescribing can have potentially substantial sustainability as well as financial benefits.

Reducing unnecessary prescribing not only reduces the carbon impact from the drugs itself but can also influence people's health seeking behaviour. By giving information instead of a prescription, patients may be less likely to return for a prescription the next time they develop a simple cold [28]. This has an added benefit of environmental sustainability from reduced medicine use, reduced travel and reduced health service use. So clinicians can, in many cases, reassure patients that antibiotics are not needed because they are unlikely to improve their symptoms – and that they may also lead to unwanted adverse effects. In addition, antibiotics also increase the risk of antimicrobial resistance [29]. However, from a parental view, cough is not a trivial illness and many parents worry if their child's cough has not settled after 5–7 days. For this reason it is worth pointing out the expected duration and natural history of a symptom, as, for example, a cough due to a simple cold may last for up to four weeks [30].

Where systems are available to rank pharmaceuticals according to their environmental impact (such as in Sweden), health professionals and patients have the opportunity to make an informed choice towards less harmful medicines [31]. Prescribing advisers (where available) can help clinicians with updating and optimising their prescribing practices [32].

Avoiding medicine waste

Lack of medication adherence is a huge problem worldwide, with up to half of prescribed and dispensed drugs never being taken [33]. Disposing of unused medicines has environmental implications, such as the harmful

Box 5.1   Advice given by the High Field Surgery in Leeds (UK) to patients to reduce medicine waste (Data from [35])

- Only order what you need.
- Let your GP or pharmacist know if you've stopped taking any of your medicines.
- Check what medicines you still have at home before re-ordering.
- Discuss your medication with your pharmacist or GP on a regular basis. A confidential medicines check-up with your pharmacist will help you find out more about your medicines, identify any problems and help you take your medicines in the best way.
- Think carefully before ticking all the boxes on your repeat prescription forms and only tick those you really need.
- If you don't need the medicine, don't order it! If you need the medicine in the future you can still request it.
- If you need to go into hospital, please take all your medicines with you.
- Please remember your medicines are prescribed for you. It is not safe to share them.

impact from chlorofluorocarbons in inhalers (now being phased out in many countries) on the ozone layer [34]. Possible strategies for reducing unused, repeat prescriptions and avoiding medicine waste include:

- Aligning drug quantities for patients on multiple medications.
- Avoiding polypharmacy.
- Consider making use of registered prescribing advisers where available.
- Avoiding repeat prescriptions for drugs unless they have been shown to benefit the patient.
- Monitoring patients' medication usage and review this regularly.
- Involving patients in decisions about their medicines.

Making patients aware of medication waste is equally important. Box 5.1 shows an example of information that may be displayed in patient waiting areas, or provided when issuing prescriptions.

Using herbal medicines and other complementary therapies

Evidence shows that herbal medicines can be effective in treating various medical symptoms and conditions, such as depression or irritable bowel conditions [36, 37]. If a herbal preparation is clinically effective it will normally provide a low carbon alternative to any equivalent pharmaceutical product. This is because herbal medicines do not contain petroleum-based ingredients and require relatively little industrial processing. Although at present herbal products do often travel long distances to market and are not always sustainably sourced (for example, some wild plant populations, such as ginseng and Echinacea, have suffered from excessive collection, and some popular plant remedies still travel great distances to their destination) there is at least the potential to grow useful herbs close to where they will be needed [38]. Many herbal remedies are abundant in the wild (and/or can be easily cultivated), so can often play a role as low-cost and low-carbon sustainable alternatives to highly manufactured medicines. Perhaps in the future we will see the reappearance of the *physic garden* as a source of medicinal plants and community education [39].

Compared to typical conventional interventions, complementary medicine usually has a considerably lower carbon impact. Something such as massage requires no more than a warm room. However, sustainability is only one of our measures of quality and complementary therapies also need to effective, affordable and accessible. Good quality clinical trials have shown specific complementary therapy interventions, such as acupuncture-point stimulation for the management of chemotherapy-induced nausea and vomiting, to be effective [40]. Others, like homeopathy and chiropractic, remain mired in controversy while researchers grapple with the methodological challenges. Complementary therapies fill a need for treatments that involve a caring unhurried therapeutic relationship and focus on wellbeing, resilience and symptom relief. Some *therapies*, such as mindfulness and Alexander Technique, are in fact *training* in self-help. As a group, complementary therapies may provide important lessons for making mainstream healthcare more holistic. *Integrative medicine* is the name of this movement pioneered in North America, which seeks to weave the best of conventional, complementary and lifestyle-based interventions into a coherent system [41, 42].

'Leaner' service delivery

When health services become more efficient, increased sustainability is often a welcome side-effect. Increasing efficiency is all about changing current ways of working: working faster, with less effort and less resources while maintaining, or – even better – improving effectiveness and quality of care. Efficiency savings and improvements can be achieved in any health system, even those that may think of themselves as advanced [8]. The *NHS Institute for Innovation and Improvement's 'Productive Series'* (www.institute.nhs.uk), for example, demonstrates that clinical teams can often create extra time

---

Case study 5.2   More efficient working practices

The Northumbria Health Care NHS Foundation Trust set up work streams to reduce the number of cancelled operations and make overall care more efficient. For example, channelling patients into pre-assessment consultations directly from clinic (rather than them going home and returning at a later date) reduced the steps in the patient journey. And informing theatre staff one week in advance of the type of surgery needed helped to optimise equipment and kit management. A last-minute weekly reminder helped to overcome the trend of patients becoming complacent about their operation date and time, which previously had led to missed slots. Their efficiency drive not only reduced the steps in the patient journey but the hospital also managed to reduce cancellations by about 50% and halve the number of patient journeys – with obvious co-benefits.

---

through surprisingly simple measures, which also improve quality of care at a reduced cost [43, 44]. Experience from the *Productive Series* is mounting that adapting techniques from efficiency drives used in car manufacturing and safety processes from the aviation industry can effectively improve health services [9]. Reducing the number of steps in current care pathways (whether these are in surgery, anaesthesia, general practice or district nursing) is often a good and easy starting point and an area where we can see benefits almost instantly [44]. For example, follow up visits (such as blood pressure monitoring) are often scheduled more frequently than necessary; reducing the number of these monitoring visits that are not clinically necessary benefits patients, finances and the environment.

To have lasting and positive effects, any such changes need to be implemented carefully and their rationale communicated clearly to everyone involved. What is important is that the people affected by the change believe in it and become a true partner in the implementation. Ideally, they become the main drivers for the change, which then becomes long-lasting, effective and positive. The results in terms of resource savings, reducing waste and improving staff morale in various healthcare settings are often impressive (Case study 5.2) [43].

As the preceding examples demonstrate, reviewing the way in which we coordinate and integrate patient care can reduce unnecessary travel and healthcare use. This is particularly relevant for specialist services which share a common patient base, such as diabetes, cardiovascular and renal care. More judicial use of diagnostic tests, such as blood tests, scans and X-rays, may lead to streamlining pathways and saves on the number of interventions; it also means that patients do not have to return on different occasions for each test [11]. Similarly, providing healthcare closer to home may not only lead to clinical and financial benefits but also carries important sustainability implications (Chapter 7) [45].

Committing health service resources sustainably

Commissioners of care often have huge power and carry great responsibilities, as they make decisions that may have immediate as well as long-lasting consequences for the communities they serve – both for patient care and environmental sustainability [46–48]. A whole systems approach and understanding local population need can help identify better and more sustainable ways of commissioning and providing patient care. This process is essential for procuring resources effectively, evaluating service quality and outcomes, and benchmarking organisational activity against similar organisations within a health system (Figure 5.1) [49].

Lower carbon communication

With rising fuel prices, the costs of transporting patients or staff will become more expensive. Consequently, in many clinical situations where patients or health professionals have to travel, using electronic communications such as

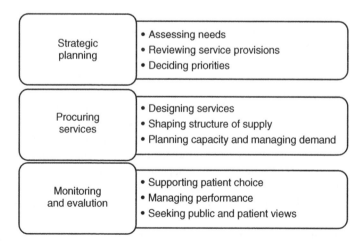

Figure 5.1 Supporting commissioning through the commissioning cycle. (Data from [49].)

online records, email and telephone can help reduce travel-related emissions (Chapter 6 gives more detail on sustainable transport). The emphasis should be on access to care: transporting patients and health professionals is one way of doing this – but not always the best by any means. Although effective means of electronic communication in terms of tele-healthcare (such as the telephone or video consultations) already exist in many settings, they are not yet widely used. This is partly because healthcare professionals and patients alike may find the use of tele-technology difficult to accept as a suitable alternative to face-to-face consultations. Perceived safety and technology issues as well as sometimes perverse financial incentives within the payment system (for instance those that reward face-to-face consultations more than other forms of care) may also play a role, particularly in hospital settings. But where people have overcome this attitude, results have been encouraging (Case study 5.3).

Information and communication technology (ICT) is likely to become much more important for delivering more sustainable healthcare in the future. Yet we need to remember that electronic media also carry a carbon cost. A typical year of incoming email leads to around 135 kg CO_2e per year (which is equivalent to driving about 200 miles in an average car), and carbon emissions from the world's data centres (from powering computers and keeping them cool) already produce around 130 million tonnes of CO_2e [12]. Although the use of electronic media is by no means 'zero

---

Case study 5.3 Improving access through better use of the telephone

The 'Doctor First' programme is a way of working that aims to improve patient access through advanced telephone conversations directly with a general practitioner [50]. Tested in 41 practices in the East of England, patients benefited from easy access to a doctor, and doctors were able to control their workload better. In addition, attendances at Accident & Emergency departments were around 20% lower in the participating practices, with reductions in emergency admissions by around 8%. Apart from financial savings and clinical benefits, reduced travel and resource use means that this new way of working also carries sustainability gains. Early data suggest that remote healthcare technologies may reduce the number of emergency admissions to hospital among patients with certain long-term conditions, such as chronic obstructive pulmonary disease (COPD) [51].

Case study 5.4   Sustainability actions in high-technology areas [52]

The Queen Margaret Hospital Renal Unit in Dunfermline has reduced its use of unnecessary bags of normal saline together with priming sets and drainage bags that it kept for emergency infusion during haemodiafiltration, since sterile substitution fluid for infusion is available from a newer haemodiafiltration machine. This saved direct and indirect costs of £18 594 per year and reduced emissions by an estimated 5.3 tonnes of CO_2e per year – without any cost for implementation and no added risk to patients.

---

carbon', it will in many instances be preferable when it comes to avoiding carbon-intensive travel.

Using treatments and technologies with lower environmental impact

When assessing new and innovative medical technologies for use in clinical care, sustainability measures should always be included in their evaluation. This will help clinicians, service planners and patients to choose those treatments that are clinically effective and at the same time have the best environmental profile [10, 11]. Renal medicine is an example of a high-technology clinical field with a wide scope for increasing sustainability within clinical care (Case study 5.4).

Further details and additional case studies highlighting the sustainability opportunities in renal medicine are available on the *Green Nephrology Resource Page* [52].

Educating and empowering patients

Various ways exist to give people more knowledge and more say in their care. Some of these are not only good for health but also have environmental and financial benefits. Health promotion and preventive medicine are more effective if they fall on 'fertile ground', that is, an adequate level of *health literacy*, defined by the World Health Organization (WHO) as 'the cognitive and social skills which determine the motivation and ability of individuals to gain access to, understand and use information in ways which promote and maintain good health' [53]. Unfortunately, poor health literacy is still common. A recent systematic review of 111 studies in different settings and persons of all ages suggests that low levels of health literacy lead, among other things, to poorer health outcomes, increased mortality and people not accessing health services appropriately [54]. For people to make better decisions about their health, they need to be able to access health information effectively and make use of this information while supported by health professionals. Health systems can make a real difference in this area by giving people useful and relevant information at every opportunity, and by directing them to appropriate alternative sources of information (the *NHS Choices* website, www.nhs.uk, is an example). Improving health literacy can help with moving towards truly shared decision making and redress some of the often still prevalent power imbalance between patients and the medical profession.

By promoting better basic self-assessment of symptoms and self-care at every opportunity, health professionals have a great opportunity to help people make better use of health services (Case study 5.5). In the United Kingdom, about 57 million consultations in general practice involve minor ailments, and the estimated costs in terms of resource use and health professionals' time to the NHS of patients seeing the GP for ailments that can be self-treated is around £2 billion [55]. People who are informed about their health are better equipped to manage part of their medical care themselves (with support from health professionals), so can greatly contribute to increasing sustainability [56, 57]. Responding to health data such as home blood pressure readings, making simple decisions about medication and making better use of non-prescription therapies are examples of where

---

Case study 5.5 Promoting self-care in general practice [61]

At the Bromley-by-Bow centre in East London, UK, promoting self-care is part of every aspect of patient care. The practice has recognised that good communication is crucial for encouraging people to self-care. Having redefined the doctor–patient relationship, doctors at the health centre sit alongside their patients rather than being separated by a desk, so that they can look at the computer screen and solve problems together. This makes patients aware that doctors are not infallible and encourages them to take some responsibility for managing their ailment in the future. This has improved communication and 50% of patients leave with an information prescription – a print-out with details of free services or facilities that are available, useful numbers to ring, websites to visit or even exercises or homework to do. Patients are being encouraged to try and use these resources when they develop a health problem next time.

people can easily and safely become more involved [58]. Better patient involvement can also play an important part in reducing the risk of medical complications, thus reducing pressure on healthcare providers [59, 60].

Setting an example to patients and the public

Because of their access and interaction with the general population, health professionals have an opportunity to inform and educate the wider population about the co-benefits of living in a more environmentally sustainable way – even during clinical encounters. Good entry points are healthcare interventions that have immediate co-benefits for patients, not only in terms of improving their health but also in environmental and financial terms. Bringing sustainability aspects into discussions about increasing exercise (perhaps through more active travel) or changing to a healthier diet (by moving towards a more plant-based diet) provide a chance to raise environmental awareness.

Other opportunities include public displays in waiting areas or notices on communications, such as letter heads or phone messages. Giving a good example is a good way of spreading a message, which healthcare organisations can achieve by advertising their carbon efficiency data and sustainability. Conversely, doing nothing, saying nothing and having no opinion on these issues sets a poor example – one that others may use to justify unsustainable behaviour (exactly like smoking: 'If it were dangerous, then my doctor wouldn't smoke'). The impact of clinicians travelling by bicycle to see their patients, for example, can be astonishing, sends out important public health messages – and opens up an opportunity for discussing topics around sustainability and health (Chapter 7).

Healthcare providers may also be able to reach people who do not use health services very often by approaching the local or wider media about their sustainability events or achievements. Other useful actions include encouraging people to use public transport (by providing information on bus routes or train timetables) or to travel more actively by walking or cycling should they be well enough to do so (for example, for hospital follow-ups or screening appointments).

Calling for collaborative action

Using resources sensibly and responsibly in a way that we and others can continue to benefit from them is a universal principle that rises above differences between individuals or groups of people. We cannot predict how clinical care will develop in the next few years and decades, but we can be fairly confident that it will look very different. Advances in technology, changes in the environment and the economy (in either direction), ageing populations or uncontrolled migration (and the violence it stimulates) will influence healthcare provision in the future.

Clinicians are in a unique position to not only practice low-carbon care, but also facilitate lifestyle and attitude changes in their patients. Areas where changes in behaviour can pay particular sustainability dividends are diet and exercise, prescription management, contraception and family planning, as well as end-of-life care. Improving technical effectiveness and safety can be relatively straightforward and is important, but what really needs to be on today's agenda is to add value within given budgets – and to do this sustainably.

In this chapter, we have touched upon some of these issues but will return to them and introduce others in the chapters to come. There are still more questions than answers, but 'business as usual' is clearly not an option for clinical medicine. We simply cannot afford not to act. As the case studies in this chapter illustrate, a great deal of good work is already going on, carried out with much enthusiasm and inspiration by clinical teams all over the world. We need to share best practices. Further resources and more information about innovative and effective sustainability practices can be found at the websites of the *NHS Sustainable Development Unit* (www.sdu.nhs.uk), the *Centre for Sustainable Healthcare* (www.greenerhealthcare.org), *Healthcare Without Harm* (www.noharm.org) and many other organisations with an interest in sustainable healthcare, the number of which is growing all the time.

Other useful resources

- Fit for the Future: Scenarios for low-carbon healthcare 2030. NHS Sustainable Development Unit and Forum for the Future, Sept 2009. http://www.forumforthefuture.org/files/Fit_for_the_Future_NHS_Sept09.pdf
- Sustainable Action Planning (SAP) Resource Pack for Clinical Teams. http://sap.greenerhealthcare.org/

Key points

- Lead by example and reduce your personal carbon footprint.
- Help your organisation discover its carbon footprint.
- Ensure family planning services are functioning optimally.
- Configure services to focus on health promotion.
- Give patients greater responsibility for managing their health.
- Avoid unnecessary prescriptions.

- Use lower carbon alternatives where possible, such as effective herbal medicines.
- Understand the concept of *lean service delivery*.
- Explore lower-carbon ways of connecting with patients, including tele-medicine.
- Stay focused on the triple bottom line of clinical, financial and environmental quality.
- Get involved in spearheading a movement towards carbon reduction and sustainable development.
- Take part in collective actions by health professionals – your voice is important to shape the opinions of the public, other professionals and policy makers.
- Lobby your professional organisations to create and raise awareness around sustainability.
- Join clinical commission groups and try to introduce sustainability measures whenever possible.

References

1. Charlesworth, A., Gray, A., Pencheon, D. and Stern, N. (2011) Assessing the health benefits of tackling climate change. *British Medical Journal*, **343**, d6520.
2. Stern, N. (2007) *The economics of climate change: the Stern review*. Cambridge University Press, Cambridge. 2007.
3. Maxwell, R.J. (1992) Dimensions of quality revisited: from thought to action. *Quality in Health Care*, **1**(3), 171–177.
4. Atkinson, S., Ingham, J., Cheshire, M. and Went, S. (2010) Defining quality and quality improvement. *Clinical Medicine*, **10**(6), 537–539.
5. Bunn, F., Byrne, G. and Kendall, S. (2004) Telephone consultation and triage: effects on health care use and patient satisfaction. *Cochrane Database of Systematic Reviews*(4), CD004180.
6. Beaver, K., Tysver-Robinson, D., Campbell, M. *et al.*(2009) Comparing hospital and telephone follow-up after treatment for breast cancer: randomised equivalence trial. *British Medical Journal*, **338**, a3147.
7. Pencheon, D. (2009) *How health services can act. The health practitioner's guide to climate change*. Earthscan Ltd, London.
8. Garber, A.M. and Skinner, J. (2008) Is American Health Care Uniquely Inefficient? *Journal of Economic Perspectives*, **22**(4), 27–50.
9. Kim, C.S., Spahlinger, D.A., Kin, J.M. and Billi, J.E. (2006) Lean health care: what can hospitals learn from a world-class automaker? *Journal of Hospital Medicine*, **1**(3), 191–199.

10. Centre for Sustainable Healthcare – Clinical transformation[Internet]. http://sustainablehealthcare.org.uk/clinical-transformation[accessed 11 August2011].
11. Mortimer, F. (2010) The sustainable physician. *Clinical Medicine*, **10**(2), 110–111.
12. Berners-Lee, M. (2010) *How Bad Are Bananas?: The carbon footprint of everything*. Profile Books, London.
13. Guillebaud, J. and Hayes, P. (2008) Population growth and climate change. *British Medical Journal*, **337**, a576–a576.
14. UNFPA, United Nations Population Fund–Publications: Population & Development [Internet]. http://www.unfpa.org/public/home/publications/pubs_pd [accessed 2 December 2011].
15. UNFPA, United Nations Population Fund – Population Issues [Internet]. http://www.unfpa.org/issues/ [accessed 2 December 2011].
16. Castro Martín, T. (1995) Women's education and fertility: results from 26 Demographic and Health Surveys. *Studies in Family Planning*, **26**(4), 187–202.
17. UNFPA, United Nations Population Fund –Family Planning: Reproductive Health [Internet]. http://www.unfpa.org/rh/planning.htm [accessed 2 December 2011].
18. International Conference on Population and Development (ICPD) (1994) [Internet]. http://www.un.org/popin/icpd2.htm [accessed 2 December 2011].
19. Pencheon, D. (2009) Health services and climate change: what can be done? *Journal of Health Services Research and Policy*, **14**(1), 2–4.
20. Evidence for Policy and Practice Information and Co-ordinating Centre (EPPI-Centre) –Database of promoting health effectiveness reviews (DoPHER) [Internet]. http://eppi.ioe.ac.uk/webdatabases/Intro.aspx?ID=2[accessed 11 August2011].
21. Haller, L., Hutton, G. and Bartram, J. (2007) Estimating the costs and health benefits of water and sanitation improvements at global level. *Journal of Water and Health*, **5**, 467.
22. World Health Organization/UNICEF (2010) Progress on sanitation and drinking-water: 2010 update. WHO/UNICEF, Geneva, Switzerland.
23. Tan, T., Little, P. and Stokes, T. (for the Guideline Development Group) (2008). Antibiotic prescribing for self limiting respiratory tract infections in primary care: summary of NICE guidance. *British Medical Journal*, **337**, a437.
24. NHS Sustainable Development Unit (2009) Saving Carbon, Improving Health: Carbon Reduction Strategy for England. NHS Sustainable Development Unit, Cambridge.
25. Gallagher, P., Lang, P.O., C.herubini. A. *et al.* (2011) Prevalence of potentially inappropriate prescribing in an acutely ill population of older patients admitted to six European hospitals. *European Journal of Clinical Pharmacology*, **67**, 1175–1188.
26. NHS Choices – Antipsychotic use in dementia [Internet]. http://www.nhs.uk/news/2009/10October/Pages/Antipsychotic-use-in-dementia.aspx [accessed 2 December 2011].

27. Straand, J. (1999) Elderly patients in general practice: diagnoses, drugs and inappropriate prescriptions. *A report from the More & Romsdal Prescription Study. Family Practice*, **16**, 380–388.
28. Little, P., Gould, C., Williamson, I., Warner, G., Gantley, M. and Kinmonth, A.L. (1997) Reattendance and complications in a randomised trial of prescribing strategies for sore throat: the medicalising effect of prescribing antibiotics. *British Medical Journal*, **315**(7104), 350–352.
29. Goossens, H., Ferech, M., Vander Stichele, R. and Elseviers, M. (2005) Outpatient antibiotic use in Europe and association with resistance: a cross-national database study. *Lancet*, **365**, 579–587.
30. Hay, A.D. (2003) The duration of acute cough in pre-school children presenting to primary care: a prospective cohort study. *Family Practice*, **20**(6), 696–705.
31. FASS.se –Startsida [Internet]. http://www.fass.se/LIF/home/index.jsp [accessed 1 November2011].
32. NHS Careers –Primary care pharmacist [Internet]. http://www.nhscareers.nhs.uk/details/Default.aspx?Id=889 [accessed 3 December 2011].
33. World Health Organization (2003) Adherence to Long-term Therapies: Evidence for Action. World Health Organization, Geneva, Switzerland.
34. United Nations Environment Programme – The Montreal Protocol [Internet]. http://www.unep.org/ozone/Montreal-Protocol/Montreal-Protocol2000.shtml [accessed 2 December 2011].
35. High Field Surgery – Avoid Medicines Waste [Internet]. http://www.highfieldsurgery.com/medicineswaste.html [accessed 2 December 2011].
36. Linde, K., Berner, M.M. and Kriston, L. (2008) St John's wort for major depression. *Cochrane Database of Systematic Reviews* (4):CD000448.
37. Merat, S., Khalili, S., Mostajabi, P., Ghorbani, A., Ansari, R. and Malekzadeh, R. (2010) The effect of enteric-coated, delayed-release peppermint oil on irritable bowel syndrome. *Digestive Diseases and Science*, **55**(5), 1385–1390.
38. Mills, S. (2011) Herbal medicines for sustainable health care. *Journal of Holistic Healthcare*, **8** (11), 43–47.
39. Jane Perrone (2011) A visit to the Urban Physic Garden. *The Guardian* [Internet]. http://www.guardian.co.uk/lifeandstyle/gardening-blog/2011/jul/28/urban-physic-garden [accessed 26 February 2012].
40. Ezzo, J.M., Richardson, M.A., Vickers, A. *et al.*(2006) Acupuncture-point stimulation for chemotherapy-induced nausea or vomiting. *Cochrane Database of Systematic Reviews* (2):CD002285.
41. May, J. (2011) What is integrative health? *British Medical Journal*, **343**, d4372.
42. Maizes, V., Rakel, D. and Niemiec, C. (2009) *Integrative medicine and patient-centered care. Explore (NY)*, **5** (5), 277–289.
43. NHS Institute for Innovation and Improvement–The Productive Series [Internet]. http://www.institute.nhs.uk/quality_and_value/productivity_series/the_productive_series.html [accessed 3 August 2011].

44. Sustainable Operating Theatres [Internet].http://sustainablehealthcare.org.uk/ sustainable-operating-theatres/feed [accessed 31 October 2011].
45. UK Department of Health –Our health, our care, our say [Internet]. http://web archive.nationalarchives.gov.uk/+/dh.gov.uk/en/healthcare/ourhealthourcare-oursay/index.htm[accessed 12 August2011].
46. NHS Sustainable Development Unit (2011)Sustainable Development for Clinical Commissioning Groups. [Internet].http://www.sdu.nhs.uk/publications-resources/67/Sustainable-Development-for-Clinical-Commissioning-Groups/ [accessed 27 November 2011].
47. NHS Sustainable Development Unit – Commissioning for Sustainability [Internet]. http://www.sdu.nhs.uk/publications-resources/8/Commissioning-for-Sustainability-/ [accessed 22 October 2011].
48. Royal College of General Practitioners – RCGP Centre For Commissioning [Internet]. http://commissioning.rcgp.org.uk/ [accessed 22 October 2011].
49. The NHS Information Centre – Support commissioning [Internet]. http://www.ic.nhs.uk/commissioning [accessed 22 October 2011].
50. East Midlands Strategic Health Authority – Rapid Telephone Access to your GP [Internet]. http://www.emqo.eastmidlands.nhs.uk/welcome/quality-indicators/care-pathways/primary-care/doctor-first/ [accessed 12 August2011].
51. Vickers, H. (2011) Telemedicine may cut emergency admissions for COPD. *British Medical Journal*, **342**, d1499.
52. Centre for Sustainable Healthcare – Green Nephrology (Resources)[Internet]. http://sustainablehealthcare.org.uk/nephrology-resources[accessed 12 August2011].
53. World Health Organization (1998) Health Promotion Glossary. World Health Organization, Geneva, Switzerland.
54. Berkman, N.D., Sheridan, S.L., Donahue, K.E., Halpern, D.J. and Crotty, K. (2011) Low health literacy and health outcomes: an updated systematic review. *Annals of Internal Medicine*, **155**(2), 97–107.
55. Proprietary Assocation of Great Britain (PAGB)(2009) Reducing GP consultations for minor ailmentswould result in significant savings & reduceddemand on the NHS (Cited from: Making the case for the self care of minor ailments, p. 5). http://www.pagb.co.uk/publications/pdfs/Minorailmentsresearch09.pdf.
56. Nielsen-Bohlman, L., Panzer, A.M. and Kindig, D.A. (eds) (2004) *Health Literacy: A Prescription to End Confusion*. National Academies Press, Washington, DC.
57. Bandura, A. (1997) *Self-efficacy: The Exercise of Control*. W.H.Freeman & Co Ltd.
58. Williams, M.V., Baker, D.W., Parker, R.M. and Nurss, J.R. (1998) Relationship of functional health literacy to patients' knowledge of their chronic disease. A study of patients with hypertension and diabetes. *Archives of Internal Medicine*, **158**(2), 166–72.
59. Wikler, D. (2002) Personal and Social Responsibility for Health. *Ethics & International Affairs*, **16**, 47–55.

60. Richardson, G., Sculpher, M., Kennedy, A. *et al.* (2006) Is self-care a cost-effective use of resources? Evidence from a randomized trial in inflammatory bowel disease. *Journal of Health Services Research &Policy*, 11(4), 225–30.

61. Self Care Forum–Case studies [Internet]. http://www.selfcareforum.org/?page_id=49 [accessed 29 November 2011].

62. Royal College of General Practitioners –Carbon footprint calculator [Internet]. http://www.rcgp.org.uk/professional_development/carbon_footprint_calculator.aspx [accessed 22 October 2011].

Chapter 6 **Food for people and planet**

In this chapter

- A short history of the western diet
- Food and human health
- Food and the global environment
- Better choices in healthy eating
- Talking food with healthcare users
- Sustainable food policy

In this chapter we look at the role that food plays in sustainable healthcare. Few topics can depict the challenges ahead so vividly. What we eat and how we produce what we eat has a profound impact on our health and the health of the planet. These two aspects can be illustrated in the illness experience of a fifty-year-old man (Box 6.1); his story is of our making, but its elements are typical of our times.

Ravi is one of the billion people on earth suffering from calorific over-nutrition while at the same time another billion people are involuntarily hungry [1]. Has food fed Ravi's health crisis? And could this same food have contributed to that other catastrophe, the inundation of the farm in Pakistan, when we know that the agricultural enterprise is responsible for one third of our global greenhouse gas (GHG) emissions? These are the central questions of this chapter. In it we look at the recent history of the Western diet and judge its contribution to the diseased heart and other ailments. And, staying faithful to a whole systems view, we consider how modern agriculture and food retailing are contributing to our global ills, especially through their intimate dependence on fossil fuels. Having rehearsed these arguments, we introduce some ideas for turning things around in the relationship between food, health and the environment, mindful of a rich seam of opportunity for establishing virtuous cycles (Chapter 3).

Sustainable Healthcare, First Edition. Knut Schroeder, Trevor Thompson, Kathleen Frith and David Pencheon.

Box 6.1   A modern scenario

Ravi lies in a modern Western hospital hypnotised by his heart trace, a visual proof that he has survived a week in which a coronary thrombosis left him on the threshold of a traumatic death. His life was likely saved by an emergency angioplasty. He feels weak and fearful but glad to be alive. Ravi has a lot on his mind. Just the week before his family in Pakistan suffered tragedy when the family homestead and farm were inundated in a flood that saw three adults and all their livestock swept away. He lifts the lid on the hospital meal and thinks, for the first time since this calamity, that he might enjoy food again. Home this afternoon, he has been talked through a small pharmacopoeia of medicines and given advice on diet and exercise. At 17 stones in weight, he needs it. Ravi is one of the 30% of citizens who live with obesity, a major risk factor for myocardial infarction.

What we have to say may be common knowledge to the initiated, but food as a topic hardly features on the menu of traditional medical and nursing education. Students learn about the nutritional components of the balanced meal and the effects of various deficiencies, but they are often starved of information on, for example, the role of the food industry, how to encourage good food practices, the pleasures – and perils – of different 'diets' and the impact of the various dietary components, such as trans-fatty acids, on health. Few medical schools teach on the global aspects of the food system. This lack of dietary detail is reflected in our medical institutions, where issues around food provision receive little attention – and often only in the most general terms. Ravi might, for instance, be invited to adhere to a low-fat diet, but many physicians will be leaving the task of curtailing cholesterol to the concomitant prescription of a lipid-lowering statin. We need a revolutionary re-education about the role that food can play in the health of both people and planet, guiding us in our transition to sustainable healthcare. We begin that re-education with the story of how we got into our current dietary difficulties.

A brief history of the 'Western Diet'

Until about 10 000 years ago, *homo sapiens* was believed to be mainly a hunter-gatherer, with a diet based principally on plants and showing little evidence of cultivation or animal husbandry. Since Neolithic times (around 10 000 BCE), mankind has engaged in agricultural practices that heralded the development of urban civilization. Food production remained broadly stable until the colonial period (starting in the 1550s) when change was spurred by maritime trade and industrialisation. An illustrative commodity is sugar. Its average consumption in the United Kingdom rose from four pounds (lbs) (1.8 kg) per head in 1700 to 18 lbs (8.2 kg) in 1800, 36 lbs (16.3 kg) in 1850 and over 100 lbs (45.4 kg) by the twentieth century. These trends mirror an expansion in trade and industrial processing. Ravi, judging by US figures, could consume 200 lbs (90.7 kg) of sugar per year – most of it embedded in processed food; sales of bagged sugar have actually fallen [2].

The most profound changes to the global diet have come in the period since 1945 with what was termed, in the 1960s, the *Green Revolution*. This combined commercial zeal, scientific research and governmental policy to create a huge increase in production capacity. It was a 'bold new programme' (Henry Truman, 1949), using artificial fertilisers, pesticides, advanced irrigation techniques and improved strains. Production of cereals doubled between 1961 and 1985. These post-war changes succeeded in bringing calorific sufficiency to millions and were associated with increased height, weight and life expectancy across the globe [3].

In systems terms, the failure of the Green Revolution was to judge its success by too simple a metric, focusing on the *quantity* of food produced and underplaying the importance of quality and environmental impact. Alongside the Green Revolution we also had a revolution in the processing of primary foodstuffs. Processed food is much easier to store and, therefore, retail than fresh food (which is one of the reasons why small local food stores often do not stock much fresh produce). It can also be branded, marketed and manipulated to satisfy our genetic predilection for fat, sugar and salt. Processed food is faster to buy, cook (or simply heat) and eat. The fuse of the Green Revolution was ignited by the increasing availability of cheap oil upon which all aspects of food production are heavily dependent.

So this is the nutritional milieu in which Ravi has grown up. He is of South Asian descent. He has been back to his village in Pakistan and eaten its traditional cuisine: freshly cooked rice, spices, pulses, mutton and vegetables. But Ravi, now a taxi driver in a big city, has adopted a distinctly Western lifestyle and diet that he fits around his working day. What is the evidence that his diet, which includes daily fast-food eaten in his cab, has contributed to his arterial calamity?

Food and human health

The links between what we eat and our health have been observed since antiquity. Good nutrition was, for instance, a foundational element of Hippocratic medicine from which canon comes the dictum 'our food should be our medicine and our medicine should be our food'. Nutrition as scientific endeavour and as popular culture is a huge enterprise. Despite the core elements of healthy eating being relatively simple and uncontested (as discussed later in this chapter), the field is fraught with contradictory information and many different diets, plans and programmes, often muddled up with commercial interests. Even *bona fide* university-based nutritional research faces many challenges. For example, getting volunteers to make meaningful dietary changes for long enough to observe the effects on health outcomes such as heart disease and cancer is difficult. More often we have to rely not on such experimental studies but on associations between lifestyle changes and health that are less robust. But despite this uncertainty, a clinically useful consensus on the elements of healthy eating is emerging. This book is not the place to review the links between diet and health; instead we consider three sentinel conditions: obesity, diabetes and cancer.

Obesity

Ravi's obesity is an obvious place to start. Projections for the United Kingdom show that for males aged 40–65, a concerning 44% will be clinically obese by 2020 [4]. In the United States, the world's most adipose country, nearly one third of all adults (around 70 million people) are already obese. And it is not only adults who are getting heavier. According to the *US Centre for Disease Control (CDC)*, the prevalence of obesity in US children aged 6–11 has tripled over a period of 30 years and lay at 20% in 2008, with serious consequences for mental and physical health [5]. Such children can look forward to an increased likelihood of diabetes, hypertension, heart disease, arthritis, certain cancers, sleep apnoea and to experiencing low self-esteem. In the process, these heavier US citizens in 2006 consumed an estimated $117 billion (£73 billion) in attributable health costs. If Ravi had been admitted in the United Kingdom, his treatment would have cost the National Health Service (NHS) around £7000 (US$ 11 300). The obesity epidemic is beginning to add up to a sustainability catastrophe – and not only in richer countries. We can also see marked rises in obesity (and its consequent health problems) in many lower-income countries and fast-growing economies, including Pakistan and China [6].

Diabetes

There is a high probability that Ravi will one day also have to learn to live with Type 2 diabetes, a condition that shows a similar morbidity pattern to obesity and has a high prevalence in South Asians. Already a quarter of Americans over 65 are diabetic. The World Health Organization (WHO) estimates that the worldwide prevalence will *double* between 2005 and 2030 and, again, there is a worrying trend for the emergence of Type 2 diabetes in the young. We are all aware of the numerous negative health impacts of diabetes, particularly on heart, kidney and eye disease. No one is denying the rocketing trends in prevalence for obesity and diabetes, but are these pandemics actually *caused* by our diet [7]?

Cancer

In the case of the cancer diagnosis, aetiological research has been exhaustively synthesised by the *World Cancer Research Fund (WCRF)* in its 2007 report [8]. The WCRF concludes that a full one third of cancers could be avoided by a move towards the non-refined whole food diets we describe later. Cancers of the gastrointestinal (GI) tract are especially influenced by dietary factors, with processed meats being a particular culprit [9]. Dietary factors are also believed to contribute to the high incidence of the hormone dependent tumours of breast, prostate and ovary in the West [10].

Proving the link

Because changes in our diets co-exist with lots of other cultural features, it is difficult to prove the links between whole diets and disease apart from a few specific associations, like those reported with cancer. Multiple studies have shown that traditional cultures, with very diverse gastronomies, have comparatively low levels of obesity, diabetes and heart disease [11]. People from these non-industrial societies are prone to the negative effects of the Western lifestyle when they encounter it. But the process is mutable. Australian researchers were able to reverse trends in obesity, hypertension and hyperlipidaemia in a small cohort of Aboriginal bushman after seven weeks of returning to their traditional diet and pastimes [12]. Dietary interventions can also prevent Type 2 diabetes as described later in this chapter. The overall evidence strongly suggests that what we eat is a significant component of the pathogenic capacity of the Western lifestyle.

Ravi eats a fast-food meal most days; he likes fries, he likes to add salt and he loves cakes and biscuits. So his diet has probably contributed to his heart attack – and to the levels of obesity and heart disease prevalent in Western societies. Ravi may never have thought about this before but since he is keen to get well again he might start to take a keener interest in what and how much he eats, especially if he gets the right guidance. The post-war Green Revolution has been a mixed blessing in terms of human health. Ravi is of South Asian cultural heritage and though living in the West is personally touched by another major factor - the impact of our food systems on the health of the planet. Three members of his extended family were swept to their deaths in the Pakistan floods of 2010 and the family farm remains waterlogged and unproductive. It is to this aspect of the story to which we now turn our attention.

Food and the global environment

According to the definitions offered in Chapter 3, eating well is a cornerstone of human resilience, providing us with immeasurable nutritional and social benefits. But food arrives on the supermarket shelf with a complex history that often impacts negatively on a global environment that is already creaking under the burden of our dietary demands (Figure 6.1).

Fossil fuels

Modern agriculture depends on a plentiful supply of fossil fuels. The presence of these exogenous hydrocarbons in the food chain is one of those 'invisible

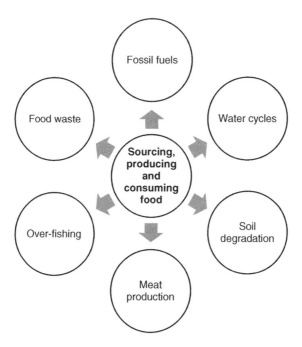

Figure 6.1 Environmental impacts of food sourcing, production and consumption.

parts' discussed in Chapter 3. According to the *US Department of Agriculture*, on average 10 kJ of fossil fuel energy are invested in the production of 1 kJ of food energy for consumption. This means that even our low-fat food is largely made of oil. Consider also how an estimated 50% of the earth's population rely on ammonium-based fertilisers for its existence, made by combining hydrogen from natural gas with atmospheric nitrogen in the Haber–Bosch process; in 2006 an estimated 147 million tonnes of ammonia were thus synthesised. Traditional methods of crop rotation are often deemed no longer necessary, as soil deficiencies are rectified by exogenous chemicals. Fossil fuels also form the chemical basis of herbicides and pesticides, which are essential for maintaining yields in bountiful but pest-sensitive food plant varieties. The inventory continues with oil needed for farm equipment, haulage, processing, packaging and the various aspects of retail, including refrigeration and consumer transport. Researchers have carried out exacting analyses of the energy invested in food production, with often sobering results. For instance, it takes about 3600 kcal (15 MJ) of energy to produce a typical cheeseburger, whilst its nutritional content is around 400 kcal [13]. A cheeseburger, then, consumes nine times the energy it delivers – the true 'cost' of a cheap burger.

Impacts on water cycles

According to the United Nations, one fifth of the world population is short of water, a figure exacerbated by climate change (Chapter 2). As our population grows, the amount of water consumed per person increases even faster and has tripled in the last 50 years. Agriculture contributes to these shortages by importing water from rivers, lakes and aquifers in competition with the demands of industry and domestic consumers. Analysts expect water scarcity to be a greater threat to global security than fuel shortages, because though we have lived without oil for most of our evolution, we cannot live without water [14]. This is particularly the case in the basins of Africa's Nile, Niger, Volta and Zambezi rivers. Egyptian agriculture depends almost wholly on the Nile, but the waters are so exploited that it hardly makes it to the sea during the dry season. The Nile flows through Ethiopia, Sudan and Egypt, which had a combined population of 195 million in 2010. As the population grows, to, for instance, a predicted 350 million by 2050, the water stress of the region will become increasingly acute and could spark conflict [15]. Industrial agriculture also impacts on the *quality* of our waters. The nitrogen-rich compounds found in fertiliser run-offs enhance the growth of marine phytoplankton leading to aquatic oxygen depletion [16]. There is, for instance, a dead zone covering 6000 square miles at the mouth of the Mississippi in the Gulf of Mexico, struggling to support the usual oceanic fauna [17]. This problem is also true of half the lakes in the United States. Fossil fuel mediated global warming also affects agriculture directly through its effects on precipitation (Chapter 2) and was the probable cause of the floods of 2010 in Pakistan (that claimed lives and livelihoods in Ravi's family) and other recent droughts and floods [18].

Soil dissociation

Rather like a breakfast cereal which compensates for the lack of natural whole grain with added nutrients, the soils of industrial agriculture are also denuded and depend on the addition of exogenous fertilisers. Soil is a complex, structured and water-retaining mix of organic and mineral matter. While it takes thousands of years to form (estimated at one inch per 750 years), it can easily be destroyed within a few years. The Earth's soil is also threatened by fertilisers whose anions acidify the soil and by the precipitation of acidic rain. In addition, deforestation and over-grazing compromise the soil structure and make it prone to erosion. For instance, each year 1.6 billion tonnes of sediment pass down China's Yangtze River from the Loess Plateau, making desertification one of the country's most pressing environmental concerns. Coastal soils are also at risk of salination where aquifers are over-exploited.

Meat production

Meat production is so problematic that it deserves a section of its own. The global market for meat is expanding rapidly, despite its production being extravagantly carbon-intensive and its consumption, especially when processed, being both hyper-calorific and carcinogenic. Meat consumption in the United States and Europe has been uniformly high in the last fifty years, and global consumption is set to double by 2050. The current spike in demand is coming from the emerging nations' new-found taste for livestock. For example, meat consumption per person per annum in China rose from 3.8 kg in 1961 to 52.4 kg in 2002, and the Chinese already eat 50% of the world's pig meat.

The problem with meat production is its stark energy inefficiency. Whereas, by tradition, farm animals foraged for scraps or ate grass, meat production takes place increasingly in 'feed lots', large mechanised systems for turning carbohydrate into protein. A third of all grain and 90% of soya beans are used to feed animals rather than people, and a cow has to eat 16 kg of grain to produce 1 kg of beef. It is also an astonishing fact that 18% of global greenhouse gas emissions are attributable to livestock production.

So our lust for meat is associated with an intensive feedstock agriculture that is hungry for land, water and fertilisers, and plant-based feeds are often exported over long distances. China is now the world's largest soya importer and second largest importer of grains. Meat is marketed as an important means of meeting human protein needs, but the only really good reason to eat meat is because it tastes good; growing grains and pulses for protein would be much healthier for people and planet. This argument is conclusively unpacked in the UN *Food and Agriculture Organisation's (FAO)* 2006 report *Livestock's Long Shadow* [19].

A sea of trouble

Scientists predict that if we continue fishing as we are now, we will see the end of most seafood by 2048 [20]. The 2009 book and film *The End of the Line* chronicles how demand for cod off the coast of Newfoundland in the early 1990s led to the decimation of the most abundant cod population in the world, how hi-tech fishing vessels leave no escape routes for fish populations and how farmed fish as a solution to this catastrophe is a myth. According to the *World Wildlife Fund (WWF)*, our oceanic and coastal fisheries, once considered inexhaustible, are now in a state of global crisis. Overfishing threatens coastal communities and the food security of the millions who rely on marine fish as an important source of protein. According to the *Food and Agriculture Organization (FAO)*, about 70% of our global fisheries is now being fished either close to, already at, or beyond their capacity, and as many as 90% of all the oceans' large fisheries have been fished out. Again the trend is for the demise of the small and the dominance of the large. Industrialised fishing is responsible for 50% of the world's catches. And, just as most of our grain feeds animals not humans, 30% of this catch is used to make fishmeal for feeding livestock. Thankfully, sustainable fishing has found formidable friends in organisations such as the *Marine Stewardship Council (MSC)*.

Many claims have been made about the health benefits of eating oily fish, such as anchovy, herring, mackerel and sardine. For example, consumption of oily fish has been linked with enhanced cognitive development in infants, reduced risk of Alzheimer disease and dementia, and reduced risk of cardio-vascular disease [21–23]. Governments across the world have taken this on board: the UK *Food Standards Agency* recommends eating at least one portion of oily fish per week, which amounts to 140 grams when cooked. Currently the UK population consumes around 50 grams per week, but following gov-ernment recommendations would mean that consumption would increase threefold. With the world's fish resources already so depleted, this creates a dilemma for the concerned consumer. The Marine Conservation Society has produced a 'Good Fish Guide' (available at www.goodfishguide.com.uk

and as a smartphone application) which rates each species for the degree to which it is endangered. Good choices include mackerel, herring and sardines. Beneficial Omega-3 fatty acids are also available from plants in the form of hemp seeds, linseeds and walnuts, and these have been shown to confer equivalent benefits [24].

Food waste

According the UK Government sponsored website www.lovefoodhatewaste .com, the British throw out around 7.2 million tonnes of purchased edible food per annum at a cost of £680 (US$ 1095) per annum for a family of four. The carbon used to produce that wasted food is equivalent to that used by a quarter of the nation's cars. Cooking more than can be consumed and not using food in time are cited as the two main reasons for this waste. At a time of global food poverty and ecological stress this is a senseless waste of resources. In 2011, the FAO sponsored a major study of food waste which concluded that about *one third* of the food produced in the world for human consumption (around 1.3 billion tonnes) gets lost or wasted every year. Not only is the food itself wasted but so are the resources used in its production [25].

Health services spend an enormous amount of energy, money and carbon to bring food and drink to the table for patients, staff and visitors. Unfortunately, this can sometimes be a futile effort. In the United Kingdom alone, an estimated 13 million patient meals ended up untouched or unserved in 2005–2006 [26]. This amasses to around £18 million (US$ 29 million) in food costs, rising to £144 million (US$ 230 million) if food preparation and staff costs are also included [27]. Because of fluctuations in demand it is impossible to avoid food waste entirely, but responsive systems which, for instance, cancel meals for patients who need to stay 'nil by mouth', can minimise waste without compromising on quality.

In this section on food and the global environment two additional themes are considered that illustrate the social and political implications of our current system: the health of agriculture workers and food security.

Health of agricultural workers

Agricultural work has been described by the *International Labour Organization* as one of the three most hazardous occupations (together with construction and mining) [28]. An estimated 170 000 agricultural workers are killed each year. Millions more farmers and workers are seriously injured by machines, suffer musculoskeletal disorders and endure ill health from environmental pathogens and agricultural pesticides. The *USA National Cancer Institute* adds leukaemia, non-Hodgkin lymphoma, soft tissue sarcoma and cancer of the stomach, brain and prostate to the list of diseases that show a higher incidence among farming communities [23]. Farmers are also often the first to bear the brunt of the effects of a drought or flood, as we saw in Pakistan in 2010. Long-term droughts, combined with mounting debts, have been blamed for the 200 000 suicides since 1997 among farmers in India [29]. To maintain a basic level of health for themselves and their families, it is critical that poor farmers are paid a guaranteed minimum price for their produce, with a margin built in to allow for development in education and healthcare. This is just what is being successfully promoted and achieved by the *Fairtrade* movement: according to the www.fairtrade.co.uk website, consumers spent £1.6 billion worldwide on Fairtrade certified products in 2007.

Food security

Food security is usually defined as physical and economic access to food that meets people's cultural preferences and nutritional needs. World food prices shot up in 2007 and 2008 due to a combination of droughts in grain-producing countries and rises in oil prices (and hence the cost of fertilisers and transport). More than 20 countries across Africa and Asia saw food-related riots, and the government of Haiti was forced to resign [30]. We have a situation where food prices will likely continue to increase as demand for food grows and production capacity reaches its limit or even starts to fall. In this inflationary environment any severe crop failure, due to drought or disease, in one of the world's main grain producing countries would have profound ramifications for the food security of the world's poorest and most vulnerable, including the 850 million people who are already chronically hungry. This is just what happened in 2006 when drought-related crop failure caused Australia's annual wheat production to drop from 25 million tonnes to 9.8 million tonnes, contributing to the 2007 spike in global food prices.

So food is not a neutral agent in the world but something with a huge impact on the global system. In this chapter we have explored the history of the Western diet and how it affects health and the environment. Health professionals are well placed to contribute proactively to the reversal of the negative trends that have been outlined. Here is a clear-cut example of a virtuous cycle: a healthy diet is also a sustainable diet in environmental terms and the healthcare community has a great opportunity to advocate healthy eating practices. We can do this through our personal choices, our clinical practice and by making healthy food the centre of health policy.

Putting food on the healthcare table

There are several tables to consider: our own tables with the food choices we make on a daily basis; the table in the consulting room, where food can and should form a routine part of our dialogue with patients; and the tables of our institutions, particularly our hospitals. Finally, there are the metaphorical tables of health and public policy. Take a seat at any of these tables and see what possibilities are on the menu.

Be the change

It is of course easier to change ourselves than it is to change others. Our private choices may not always be apparent to those we seek to influence, but by living the changes we seek in others we lend credibility to our own persuasive efforts. Also, because we are dealing here with virtuous cycles, we gain inspiration from observing positive outcomes in our own lifestyles. Though nutritional knowledge is vital, it also is really important to think in terms of the whole food experience. From a sustainability perspective we are interested in nutrients but we are even more interested in what we actually do with food – growing, shopping, cooking and eating it.

Growing your own

Growing food ourselves helps us to eat it in its freshest possible condition, free from pesticides and with nutrients intact. Children who grow up around home-grown food eat more vegetables and enjoy doing so [31]. Though subjects in blinded studies were unable to taste the difference between organically certified and non-organically certified foods, anecdotally, some foods, like tomatoes, are reputed to taste distinctly better [32]. Growing your own can also save money, provide exercise and a sense of achievement – and growers often report that they are less likely to waste food they have grown themselves. The garden or allotment also provides a destination for every scrap of organic kitchen waste.

Shopping for the planet

A key concept in sustainable shopping and one of the prerequisites of a resilient system is 'diversity' (as described in Chapter 3), and diversity of shops and diversity of foods in particular. With just a few major players, supermarkets are the antithesis of diversity, narrowing the range of small high street retailers and siphoning profits from local communities (between 1997 and 2002 more than 13 000 specialist stores closed around the United Kingdom). Using their market dominance, supermarkets often drive down prices, sometimes below the cost of production, and thus may perpetuate environmentally suspect practices [33]. Many of us value the convenience, range and prices of the supermarket, but the environmentally aware shopper also includes small stores and farmer's markets in their shopping repertoire.

What foods to buy?

There is a growing consensus on what constitutes a healthy diet, captured beautifully in the aphorism 'Eat Food, Mostly Plants, Not too Much' [34]. The food writer Michael Pollan considers many processed foods better described as 'edible food-like substances'. In other words, it is the processing of food that appears to be associated with the health risk. The call to eat 'food' therefore is not as banal as it sounds. For Pollan 'food' is only food when it has been made, preferably in your own home, from identifiable primary ingredients that your grandmother would probably recognise, such as fruits, roots, leaves, seeds, spices, diary, fish, and specific cuts of meat.

What foods not to buy?

The answer seems to be the ones that are heavily processed, salted, sugared, enhanced, flavoured and packaged. That is, in fact, most of the food in most local convenience stores (supermarkets, on the other hand, do stock lots of fresh food) [35]. We have seen already the WCRF speak out against processed meats. These claims are backed by recent research. For example, results from two prospective cohort studies in 2012 that followed-up 121 342 persons over 28 years showed that just under 20% of deaths could be prevented by reducing the consumption of processed red meat consumption to less than half a serving (about 42 grams) per day [36]. Processed food is also often full of unhelpful 'empty carbs', that is, carbohydrate that is low in nutrients and high in the potential to make us put on weight (as fat). Paradoxically food that is sold as 'low fat' may be off the list too. The rise in prevalence of the 'fat is bad' message coincided with the emergence of the obesity epidemic since the 1970s. In eating less fat we have not eaten fewer calories but more. The list of foods not to buy must include bottled water. There is no evidence that it is healthier, it can cost as much as petrol (gas), it generates a phenomenal amount of plastic waste, only 20% of which is recycled, and diverts municipal priorities away from domestic water systems. Finally, on the not to buy list are endangered species – which in practice means species of fish. See the MSC's www.FishOnLine.org for an up-to-date list of what is under-stocked and what is not.

Seasonable and organic foods

To maximise the sustainability of their procurement, readers must also consider how their food purchases are grown and transported. Organic food is allowed only a whiff of pesticide and artificial fertilisers are banned altogether. Organic certification also demands high standards of animal welfare and bans the routine (as opposed to therapeutic) use of antibiotics. On the farm, Organics' fossil fuel usage is 50% that of conventional farming [37]. However, in the United Kingdom you can still buy organic strawberries in winter, flown in from the tropics. The judicious shopper pays attention to the seasonality of their food to ensure minimum food mileage, though this is only one part of food's footprint. In springtime, less carbon may be generated by flying food from Spain, where it has ripened without the need for heated tunnels. The United Kingdom's creative www.eatseasonably.co.uk campaigning website has seen sign-up from many leading retailers.

Eating well together

When it comes to eating well we do not typically pay much attention to actually *eating* well. When we focus on the actual eating of food we stray far from notions of nutrition and into the complex territory of food *culture*. The where, the when, the how and the 'with whom' of eating are enshrined in regional and family (often matrilineal) tradition. The *French Paradox* illustrates this point: French people suffer a relatively low incidence of coronary heart disease and obesity, despite having a diet relatively rich in saturated fats. They also enjoy a unique gastronomic culture. The French spend more time at table, have a stronger tradition of family dining, eat more courses but smaller portions and rarely go in for 'seconds'. Drawing on this and other traditional eating cultures, Pollan offers a formula against the fallacy of fast food which is in line with the ideas of the *Slow Food* movement that emerged from Rome in the 1980s [38]: healthy eating is eating we do slowly, together, and during meals at tables – ideally not alone, not at a desk and not in front of the television. The health benefits of eating slowly are confirmed by studies showing that it takes the stomach twenty minutes to register that it is full, by which time a lot of calories can pass under the alimentary radar. In systems terms, eating slowly gives our bodies time to register feedback and to adjust.

Food in the consulting room

Readers in clinical practice may recognise that their patients are a long way from instigating the sorts of changes suggested here. Theories of behaviour change (as discussed in Chapter 3) show that people will often make changes in proportion to the perceived threat to their health. If people are reasonably healthy, the threat to their health from their diets may feel minimal. But someone like Ravi, who has just had a myocardial infarction, may be more attuned. For all the good reasons given in this chapter so far, food reform sits at the heart of sustainable healthcare. Nothing short of a revolution in our priorities is called for. This is something that all health professionals can weave into their practice. We begin by looking at some of the factors that underpin unhealthy eating choices.

Why people eat unhealthy food

Processed food products exploit our genetic tendency to crave those foods which were prized during our evolutionary past: salt, sugar and animal fat. These tastes have immediate appeal and tend to leave us wanting more. Basic processed foods are relatively cheap to buy, even if the environmental costs of their production are high. Such foods are often either ready to eat or quick to prepare. In the United States, 25% of calories are consumed in the car. A poignant scene from the film *Food, Inc.* shows how a low-income family finds supermarket vegetables unaffordable, opting instead for drive-through burgers [39]. Ironically, their food poverty is greatly exacerbated by the cost of cardiovascular prescription medicines for the father. Advertisers earn their dollars convincing people, particularly children, to eat branded, processed foods – with little regulation to stop them getting inside our heads and stomachs. In addition, the last 20 years have seen a major increase in portion sizes [40]. The complexities of food are also apparent in the emotional comfort provided by foods such as chocolate. When we aspire to help people change people's diets we are touching upon some very complex issues.

Evidence for dietary interventions

Given the powerful forces that drive bad eating habits, is it worth the effort to address these in clinical practice? Certainly in United Kingdom primary care, many health professionals are sceptical about the usefulness of obesity guidelines [41]. Yet good evidence is available for the effects of dietary modification as part of high-intensity lifestyle interventions that often include both exercise and stress reduction components. In a raft of fascinating studies, Ornish and colleagues have shown that a lifestyle regimen with a strong focus on healthy eating can lead to a reversal of coronary atherosclerosis without recourse to drugs or surgery [42]. The evidence of benefit is greater in such high risk groups. For instance, in persons with impaired glucose tolerance (IGT), diet and exercise interventions can prevent the development of diabetes. Among the 522 middle-aged subjects of the *Finnish Diabetes Prevention Study*, the cumulative incidence of diabetes after four years was 11% in the lifestyle group, and 23% in the control group [43]. The *Diabetes Prevention Programme*, again aimed at those with IGT, estimated a number-needed-to-treat of seven persons to prevent one case of diabetes, comparing favourably with pharmaceutical measures [44].

What diets to recommend

A search, in 2012, of the books section of Amazon.com, using the word 'diet' returned over 64 000 hits. How can health professionals sift through the hype and make a reasoned recommendation? Though health professionals can be scornful about diet books, they provide an important bridge between a general dictum like 'eat mainly plants' and what happens in the supermarket and in the kitchen. People need a narrative to latch onto, they need steps for moving to a healthier diet, and they need recipes. We have a reasonably steady consensus that recommended diets should be based on fresh fruits, vegetables, nuts, spices and moderate quantities of unprocessed fish, meats and diary. Many branded diets follow suit. The *DASH* diet (Dietary Approaches to Hypertension) was studied in hypertensives but is now recommended by the *US Department of Agriculture (USDA)* as an ideal eating plan for all Americans [45]. The *Mediterranean Diet* is similar but with most fats coming from olive oil. Good adherence to these diets is associated with a range of positive cardiovascular and metabolic end-points [46]. Ornish's '*Spectrum*' diet is also recommended because it has been used in formal clinical studies with positive outcomes [47]. The concept of the *glycaemic index (GI)* is relatively easy to convey in the consulting room. Foods with a high GI are those which are rapidly digested and absorbed, resulting in wider fluctuations in blood sugar levels. In contrast, low-GI foods, by virtue of their slow digestion and absorption, produce gradual rises in blood sugar and insulin levels, and have proven benefits for health [48]. The Atkin's and other low carbohydrate diets, with their emphasis on animal protein, are not recommended on sustainability grounds. We list helpful resources for further reading about diets at the end of this chapter. When it comes to recommending diets there is no substitute for the experience of learning to eat more healthily oneself. It is a convenient truth, worth repeating, that diets that are good for people are also good for the planetary system by being less processed, less centred on animal protein and more likely to be sourced locally.

Practical tips for practitioners

Across the world many people, particular young people, have come to consider highly processed and sweetened grain products, that is, 'breakfast cereals', as a necessary part of their morning regimen. This is a triumph of marketing, pioneered in nineteenth century America. These cereals are fortified with vitamins and minerals, because the nutrients in the original seeds have been lost during puffing, baking, rolling, salting, sugaring and extruding. Some contain 40% pure sugar [49]. So for breakfast promote fruit, porridge (oatmeal) and bread as healthier alternatives. Ask patients about whether they consume many sugary drinks. People often consider fruit and fruit-flavoured drinks as healthy and even part of their *five a day* regimen of fruit consumption. Thought fine in moderation, fruit drinks can also be a deceptively easy way to consume large amounts of high glycaemic index calories. To maintain an adequate fluid intake, encourage tap water and locally grown fresh fruit instead. Keep samples of things like interesting grains (millet and quinoa), seeds (linseed and hemp seeds), nuts (walnut and brazil) and simple preparation instructions available at your place of practice. An 'Eatwell Plate' can be useful for showing a visual depiction of what a healthy meal looks like on the plate, divided into the different main components [50].

Food in hospitals

It is really important to get it right with hospital food and a scandal when we get it wrong. In the United Kingdom the NHS spends £500 million per annum serving up 300 million meals. Procurement choices here can have big sustainability impacts. But, at present, formal regulations on what hospitals in the United Kingdom and the United States can serve are lacking, with sustainability typically low on the agenda. A Kings Fund report in the United Kingdom looked at the food miles of several commonly served dishes finding, for instance, that the mileage of steak (Argentinean) and kidney (New Zealand) pie was in the region of 30 000 km [51]. It seems obvious that the food in hospitals should be of the sort we have already established to be generative of good health. Hospitals could even be environments where people discover new and healthier eating practices. Imagine, for instance, if Ravi's discharge planning included cookery classes, or if his pre-discharge home visit included a look at the family shopping inventory and kitchen set-up. If not actively promoting healthy food, hospitals should at least not passively endorse unhealthy food. Yet surveys show that about 40% of academically-affiliated US hospitals contain on-site branded fast food franchises such as MacDonald's and Burger King (which boast a branch in the main concourse of Addenbrook's Hospital in Cambridge, UK) [52].

But would healthy food simply cost too much and risk straining peoples' palates when in need of comfort in a time of health crisis? Apparently not, according to some case studies of publically funded hospital catering in the United Kingdom and United States (Case studies 6.1–6.3).

With such influence in clinical environments, health professionals can do a great deal to advance the sustainability agenda. But to change the catering practices of a whole hospital or Health Maintenance Organisation (HMO),

---

Case study 6.1   Cornwall Food Programme

Since 2001, the NHS in Cornwall has pioneered an innovative approach to buying and cooking food. The *Cornwall Food Programme* is based on the idea of popular, fresh and nutritious food, sourced locally. For instance, a locally made fishcake has replaced the nationally procured version (which was allegedly 'as hard as a hockey ball'). The contracts for fruit and vegetables, meat, fresh milk, eggs and dried goods are now all awarded to Cornish companies but all still within a parsimonious budget of £2.50 (US$ 4)per patient per day. Patient feedback shows increasing satisfaction with the quality and taste of the meals, and delivery vehicle food miles have dropped by 67% [53].

Case study 6.2   Nottingham University Hospitals Trust

Here the food travels less distance than the 7000 patients who choose from the menu each day. The local NHS Trust's catering policy supports dozens of local farmers and has ploughed over £1 million (US$ 1.6 million) into the local economy. The startling finding in Nottingham is that not only is there plenty of local food about (of excellent quality) but the whole operation is costing the NHS per day less than before the farm-to-plate scheme was initiated. Nottingham provides a heartening example of what is possible with vision and committed leadership. The City Hospital sources its 1000 pints (568 litres) of milk per day from a farm 11 miles away. Meat comes mainly from local farms and fish from MSC approved sources.

Case study 6.3   The Health Food in Healthcare (HFHC) Pledge

HFHC is the leading organisation pressing for food reform in the US health sector. Launched in 2006, the HFHC Pledge provides a vehicle through which hospitals can revitalise their food practices and send an important signal to the marketplace [54]. As of August, 2011, more than 350 hospitals, health systems and long-term care facilities across 38 states had signed the Pledge. Pledged facilities range in size from 30 beds to more than 1000 beds. In a related initiative, HFHC awards *Sustainable Food Procurement Awards* to facilities such as *Fletcher Allen Health Care* in Burlington, Vermont. Fletcher Allen purchased most products from local suppliers and 35% of its meat and poultry purchases were raised without antibiotics.

---

we need to change not just people but *policy*. The word has connotations of dullness, proceduralism and regulation and the idea of changing it seems beyond the powers of most. Yet there are many inspiring examples of sustainable evolution within organisations (as above) and of revolutions wrought by individual campaigners.

Food policy for people and planet

Policy is something that can belong to organisations and even individuals. For instance a person can say 'my policy is to support small shopkeepers'. Here we look briefly at four national policy interventions that could, with the necessarily political will, bring about significant change.

Food labelling

On the whole, healthy food does not need labelling. When we eat carrots, potatoes, herring, hazelnuts, rhubarb, cream, apples and so on we can probably get by without a nutritional breakdown. Food labelling is a by-product of processing [55] and there are three regulatory aspects to address. Firstly, manufacturers make claims that food is healthy when there is no strong evidence that it is. Food that is 'low fat' is not intrinsically healthy and it should not be legal to say it is. Secondly, there is the information on the nutritional content of food. Foods in the United Kingdom and United States (though not, surprisingly, in some European countries) are routinely labelled with the energy, fat, protein, carbohydrate, fibre and sodium quantities per 100 g (or per serving). But it is doubtful whether this information means much to the average consumer, leading to ideas such as the 'traffic light' system, which, so far, has not gained much momentum [56]. Thirdly, there is the radical idea of labelling a food product (and indeed any consumer product) with an indication of the carbon cost of its production, thus enabling consumers to manage their personal carbon budgets alongside their nutritional health. This has already been introduced in the United Kingdom with products from, for example, Walker's Crisps, Tesco, British Sugar and others.

Working with industry

Smart organisations have seen where things are heading and want to work with regulators in the transition to a greener regimen (see for instance the wide range of initiatives at www.tesco.com/greenerliving/). Major retailers can take the initiative with policies aimed at lowering salt and hidden sugars and banning trans-fats altogether. Perhaps our best leverage as health professionals is through our professional organisations, which are often consulted by government and through international pressure groups such as WASH (World Action on Salt and Hypertension) [57]. Advertising of overtly unhealthy food, especially to the young, could be prohibited. Advertising (Coca Cola's budget in 2004 was $2.2 billion) does not just deflect choice, it creates demand. Governments should work with industry to ensure that the most vulnerable consumers are protected.

Hospital food policy

Statutory requirements for hospitals to serve healthy and sustainably sourced food are an urgent policy priority. Every hospital catering department should have this as its core mission, with governmental sticks and carrots to lever change. Each organisation could be required to publish information on the health of its food, its budgets and consumer satisfaction. Catering managers can visit the beacon examples and, in the United Kingdom for instance, sign up to the Soil Association's excellent 'Food for Life' catering mark scheme or, in the United States, to the HFHC's Pledge as described above [58]. To gain groundswell for such policy, patients should be encouraged to write to hospitals about their eating experiences – both the positive and the parlous. Health professionals working in hospitals are perfectly placed to get 'vocal for local'. In an enlightened move, the American Medical Association has passed a sustainable food policy encouraging the healthcare sector to serve healthy and sustainable food [59].

Food in health professional education

Given the centrality of food-related ills, we need to find a way to get more food on the curricular menu. As well as understanding the metabolism and balance of nutrients, and nutrition in special situations, practitioners need to understand the history of food, its environmental impacts and how to talk and advise about it. Interestingly, the UK's General Medical Council medical education requirements do state that students must be able to 'discuss the role of nutrition in health'. In Chapter 11, we discuss in more detail the role that higher education plays for increasing sustainability in the healthcare sector.

Summing up about food

Health professionals need to develop a new and radical vision of where food fits into the healthcare enterprise as both cause and cure of our most pressing problems – in particular that of obesity and overweight and their attendant ills. What is new here is the invitation to include in that vision the health of the planet. At an individual level we have to take care of how we grow, buy, cook and eat for a diet that is rich in largely unprocessed food with an emphasis on the seasonal and the local. As practitioners we should learn to engage patient in discussions about food and have access to good supportive materials and services. As hospital practitioners and managers we need to take an interest in what our kitchens are serving and how those servings are sourced. What we are calling for here is a revolution in government and health service policy that puts good food at the heart of the enterprise.

Selected useful resources

- Helpful information, including diet book recommendations, is available at www.glycaemicindex.com, which is run for the public by the University of Sydney.
- Though written in the cancer context, a well researched and freely downloadable short general dietary guide is produced by Penny Brohn Cancer Care in the United Kingdom [60].
- Clear instructions on 'How to Follow the Mediterranean Diet' are freely downloadable from the patient information website www.patient .co.uk.

Key actions

Person

• Grow your own.
• Shop with a range of retailers.
• Buy fewer processed foods.
• Eat mainly plants.
• Eat meats in moderation.
• Avoid bottled water.
• Opt for local, seasonal foods
• Enjoy cooking.
• Experiment with different diets.
• Enjoy eating with others.

Practice

• Target people at risk of food-related illness.
• Understand how to ask about eating.
• Give positive messages rather than list of 'don'ts'.
• Be willing to advise on specific diets.
• Keep print-outs of dietary advice to hand out.
• Have copies of diet books in your consulting room.
• Understand the concept of glycaemic index.
• Keep samples of dried foods for the uninitiated to view.
• Get familiar with the Eatwell plate.
• Sign up to 'Food for Life' (UK) and HFHC Pledge (USA) for hospital food.

Policy

• Nutritional labelling of all foods.
• Labelling to show the carbon costs of different foods (factoring food miles).
• Banning 'trans-fats' and other dangerous foods.
• Restrictions on advertising of unhealthy food (especially to vulnerable groups).
• Pressure on major food retailers to make staple foods healthier.
• Make food a more central element of healthcare education.

References

1. Gardner, G.T., Halweil, B. and Peterson, J.A. (1999) Underfed and Overfed: The Global Epidemic of Malnutrition. Worldwatch Institute, Washington, DC.
2. Abbott, E. (2010) *Sugar: A Bittersweet History*. Gerald Duckworth & Co Ltd, London
3. Fogel, R.W. (2004) *The escape from hunger and premature death, 1700–2100: Europe, America, and the Third World*. Cambridge University Press, Cambridge.
4. National Heart (2010) New obesity data paints a bleak future for adults [Internet]. http://nhfshare.heartforum.org.uk/RMAssets/NHFMediaReleases/2010/NHFMe diaRelease17Feb10.pdf [accessed 6 May 2011].
5. Dietz, W.H. (1998) Health consequences of obesity in youth: childhood predictors of adult disease. *Pediatrics*, **101** (3 Pt 2), 518–525.
6. Wang, Y., Mi, J., Shan, X., Wang, Q.J. and Ge, K. (2006) Is China facing an obesity epidemic and the consequences? The trends in obesity and chronic disease in China. *International Journal of Obesity*, **31** (1), 177–188.
7. van Dieren, S., Beulens, J.W.J., van der Schouw, Y.T., Grobbee, D.E. and Neal, B. (2010) The global burden of diabetes and its complications: an emerging pandemic. *European Journal of Cardiovascular Prevention and Rehabilitation*, **17** (Suppl 1), S3–S8.
8. World Cancer Research Fund/American Institute for Cancer Research – Policy Report [Internet]. http://www.dietandcancerreport.org/policy_report/index.php [accessed 22 April 2012]
9. Santarelli, R.L., Pierre, F. and Corpet, D.E. (2008) Processed meat and colorectal cancer: a review of epidemiologic and experimental evidence. *Nutrition and cancer*, **60** (2), 131–144.
10. McMichael, A.J. (2008) Food, nutrition, physical activity and cancer prevention. Authoritative report from World Cancer Research Fund provides global update. *Public Health Nutrition*, **11** (7), 762–763.
11. Price, W. (2010) *Nutrition and Physical Degeneration: A Comparison of Primitive and Modern Diets and Their Effects*. Benediction Classics Ltd, Oxford.
12. O'Dea, K. (1984) Marked improvement in carbohydrate and lipid metabolism in diabetic Australian aborigines after temporary reversion to traditional lifestyle. *Diabetes*, **33** (6), 596–603.
13. Carlsson-Kanyama, A. and Faist, M. (2000) Energy Use in the Food Sector: a Data Survey. AFR Report 291, Swedish Environmental Protection Agency, Stockholm, Sweden.
14. Dinar, S. (2002) Water, Security, Conflict, and Cooperation. *SAIS Review*, **22** (2), 229–253.
15. BBC (1999) Africa's potential water wars [Internet]. http://news.bbc.co.uk/1/hi/world/africa/454926.stm [accessed 12 May 2012].
16. Lal, R. (2009) Soils and Sustainable Agriculture: A Review. In: Lichtfouse, E., Navarrete, M., Debaeke, P., Véronique, S. and Alberola, C., (eds) *Sustainable Agriculture*, Dordrecht: Springer, Dordrecht, The Netherlands, pp. 15–23. [Internet].

http://www.springerlink.com/index/10.1007/978-90-481-2666-8_3 [accessed 22 April 2012].

17. *Science Daily* (2011) 2011 Gulf of Mexico "dead zone" could be biggest ever [Internet]. http://www.sciencedaily.com/releases/2011/07/110718141618.htm [accessed 22 April 2012].

18. Biello, D. (2011) Warning: Flooding Ahead. *Scientific American*, **304** (5), 16.

19. Food and Agriculture Organization of the United Nations (2006) Livestock's long shadow: environmental issues and options [Internet]. http://www.fao.org/docrep/010/a0701e/a0701e00.HTM [accessed 13 May 2011].

20. Worm, B., Barbier, E.B., Beaumont, N. *et al.* (2006) Impacts of Biodiversity Loss on Ocean Ecosystem Services. *Science*, **314** (5800), 787–790.

21. Daniels, J.L., Longnecker, M.P., Rowland, A.S. and Golding, J. (The ALSPAC Study Team) (2004) Fish intake during pregnancy and early cognitive development of offspring. *Epidemiology*, **15** (4), 394.

22. Morris, M.C., Evans, D.A., Tangney, C.C., Bienias, J.L. and Wilson, R.S. (2005) Fish Consumption and Cognitive Decline With Age in a Large Community Study. *Archives of Neurology*, **62** (12), 1849–1853.

23. Oomen, C.M., Feskens, E.J.M., Räsänen, L. *et al.* (2000) Fish Consumption and Coronary Heart Disease Mortality in Finland, Italy, and the Netherlands. *American Journal of Epidemiology*, 200 **151** (**10**), 999–1006.

24. de Lorgeril, M., Salen, P., Martin, J.-L., Monjaud, I., Delaye, J. and Mamelle, N. (1999) Mediterranean Diet, Traditional Risk Factors, and the Rate of Cardiovascular Complications After Myocardial Infarction: Final Report of the Lyon Diet Heart Study. *Circulation*, **99** (6), 779–785.

25. Gustavsson, J., Cederberg, C. and Sonesson, U. (2011) Global Food Losses and Food Waste. Food and Agriculture Organisation of the United Nations.

26. House of Commons Hansard Written Answers for 08 October 2007 (pt 0058) [Internet]. http://www.publications.parliament.uk/pa/cm200607/cmhansrd/cm071008/text/71008w0058.htm [accessed 16 September 2011].

27. NHS Confederation (2007) Taking the temperature: towards an NHS response to global warming. The NHS Confederation, London.

28. International Labour Organization (ILO) (2009) Agriculture: a hazardous work [Internet]. http://www.ilo.org/safework/info/WCMS_110188/lang--en/index.htm [accessed 25 November 2011].

29. India Together (2010) Nearly 2 lakh farm suicides since 1997 [Internet]. http://www.indiatogether.org/2010/jan/psa-suicides.htm [accessed 25 November 2011].

30. Reuters (2008) Haiti's government falls after food riots http://www.reuters.com/article/2008/04/13/us-haiti-idUSN1228245020080413 [accessed 2 December 2011].

31. Nanney, M.S., Johnson, S., Elliott, M. and Haire-Joshu, D. (2007) Frequency of Eating Homegrown Produce Is Associated with Higher Intake among Parents and Their Preschool-Aged Children in Rural Missouri. *Journal of the American Dietetic Association*, **107** (4), 577–584.

32. Basker, D. (1992) Comparison of Taste Quality Between Organically and Conventionally Grown Fruits and Vegetables. *American Journal of Alternative Agriculture*, 7 (03), 129–136.
33. Simms, A. (2007) *Tescopoly: How One Shop Came Out on Top and Why It Matters*. Constable, London.
34. Ornish, D. (2009) Mostly Plants. *The American Journal of Cardiology*, **104** (7), 957–958.
35. Pollan, M. (2009) *In Defence of Food: The Myth of Nutrition and the Pleasures of Eating: An Eater's Manifesto*. Penguin Books Ltd.
36. Pan, A., Sun, Q., Bernstein, A.M. *et al.* (2012) Red Meat Consumption and Mortality: Results From 2 Prospective Cohort Studies. *Archives of Internal Medicine*, **172** (7), 555–563. doi:10.1001/archinternmed.2011.2287.
37. Zentner, R.P., Basnyat, P., Brandt, S.A. *et al.* (2011) Effects of input management and crop diversity on non-renewable energy use efficiency of cropping systems in the Canadian Prairie. *European Journal of Agronomy*, **34** (2), 113–123.
38. Padovani, C.P.G. (2006) *Slow Food Revolution: A New Culture for Dining and Living*. Rizzoli International Publications, New York.
39. Food, Inc. (2009) Wikipedia [Internet]. http://en.wikipedia.org/wiki/Food,_Inc. [accessed 31 July 2012].
40. Diliberti, N., Bordi, P.L., Conklin, M.T., Roe, L.S. and Rolls, B.J. (2004) Increased Portion Size Leads to Increased Energy Intake in a Restaurant Meal[ast][ast]. *Obesity*, **12** (3), 562–568.
41. Turner, K.M., Shield, J.P. and Salisbury, C. (2009) Practitioners' views on managing childhood obesity in primary care: a qualitative study. *British Journal of General Practice*, **59** (568), 856–862.
42. Ornish, D., Brown, S.E., Billings, J.H. *et al.* (1990) Can lifestyle changes reverse coronary heart disease?: The Lifestyle Heart Trial. *Lancet*, **336** (8708), 129–133.
43. Tuomilehto, J., Lindström, J., Eriksson, J.G. *et al.* (2001) Prevention of type 2 diabetes mellitus by changes in lifestyle among subjects with impaired glucose tolerance. *New England Journal of Medicine*, **344** (18), 1343–1350.
44. Knowler, W.C., Barrett-Connor, E., Fowler, S.E. *et al.* (2002) Reduction in the incidence of type 2 diabetes with lifestyle intervention or metformin. *New England Journal of Medicine*, **346** (6), 393–403.
45. Sacks, F.M., Svetkey, L.P., Vollmer, W.M. *et al.* (2001) Effects on blood pressure of reduced dietary sodium and the Dietary Approaches to Stop Hypertension (DASH) diet. DASH-Sodium Collaborative Research Group. *New England Journal of Medicine*, 201 **344** (1), 3–10.
46. Kastorini, C.-M., Milionis, H.J., Esposito, K., Giugliano, D., Goudevenos, J.A. and Panagiotakos, D.B. (2011) The Effect of Mediterranean Diet on Metabolic Syndrome and its Components: A Meta-Analysis of 50 Studies and 534,906 Individuals. *Journal of the American College of Cardiology*, **57** (11), 1299–1313.
47. Ornish, D. (2008) *The Spectrum: A Scientifically Proven Program to Feel Better, Live Longer, Lose Weight, and Gain Health*. Ballantine Books, New York.
48. Thomas, D. and Elliott, E.J. (2009) Low glycaemic index, or low glycaemic load, diets for diabetes mellitus. *Cochrane Database of Systematic Reviews*, (1):CD006296.

49. Harvard School of Public Health – Breakfast Cereal Sugar Content List [Internet]. http://www.hsph.harvard.edu/nutritionsource/what-should-you-eat/cereal-sugar-list/ [accessed 12 January 2012].

50. NHS Choices – Eatwell plate [Internet]. http://www.nhs.uk/Livewell/Goodfood/Pages/eatwell-plate.aspx [accessed 12 January 2012].

51. The King's Fund (2009) Sustainable Food and the NHS [Internet]. http://www.kingsfund.org.uk/publications/sustainable_food.html [accessed 20 May 2011].

52. Lesser, L.I. (2006) Research Letter. *Journal of the American Board of Family Medicine*, **19** (5), 526–527.

53. Cornwall Food Programme – Welcome to the Cornwall Food Programme website... [Internet]. http://www.cornwallfoodprogramme.co.uk/ [accessed 20 May 2011].

54. Health care Without Harm – Healthy Food in Health Care A Pledge for Fresh, Local, Sustainable Food [Internet]. http://www.noharm.org/lib/downloads/food/Healthy_Food_in_Health_Care.pdf [accessed 20 April 2012].

55. Lawrence, F. (2004) *Not On the Label: What Really Goes into the Food on Your Plate*. PenguinBooks Ltd.

56. Pelletier, A.L., Chang, W.W., Delzell, J.E. and McCall, J.W. (2004) Patients' Understanding and Use of Snack Food Package Nutrition Labels. *Journal of the American Board of Family Practice*, **17** (5), 319–323.

57. World Action on Salt and Health (WASH) (Home) [Internet]. http://www.worldactiononsalt.com/ [accessed 30 May 2011].

58. Food for Life Partnership (Home) [Internet]. http://www.foodforlife.org.uk/ [accessed 30 May 2011].

59. PRNewswire (2009) American Medical Association Passes Resolution Supporting Sustainable Food System [Internet]. http://www.prnewswire.com/news-releases/american-medical-association-passes-resolution-supporting-sustainable-food-system-62156942.html [accessed 20 April 2012].

60. Penny Brohn Cancer Care (Home) [Internet]. http://www.pennybrohncancercare.org/ [accessed 27 May 2011].

Chapter 7 **Travel and transport: moving to better health**

In this chapter

- Reducing transport-related carbon emissions
- Adopting better and healthier ways of travelling
- Developing institutional travel plans

Transport in the health sector

Transporting people, goods and information is a core activity of any health system. In England, for example, transport causes around 16% of the National Health Services' (NHS) total carbon emissions [1]. There is much scope for the health sector to reduce travel-related carbon emissions while saving money and maintaining, or even improving, access to clinical care. The World Health Organization has identified four overarching goals of healthier transport relating to public health [2]:

1. Increasing equity through better access to goods and services.
2. Increasing physical activity through safe walking and bicycling.
3. Increasing safety and physical activity and reducing air pollution through use of mass transit/public transport.
4. Reducing deaths and disease from pollution (noise, air, water) and traffic injuries.

In addition, road infrastructure also causes social divides both systemically and at a local physical level by dividing communities. Unfortunately, travel does not yet have intrinsic value for all health policy makers, so health professionals have an important role in raising awareness in this area [3].

Sustainable Healthcare, First Edition. Knut Schroeder, Trevor Thompson, Kathleen Frith and David Pencheon.

In this chapter, we explore strategies to make health-related travel and transport more sustainable, such as reducing the need to travel, travelling more efficiently and developing institutional travel plans.

The health and carbon effects of travel and transport

According to the UK Department for Transport, cars travelled an estimated 244 billion miles on United Kingdom roads in 2010 (which roughly equates to about 12 000 miles per car per year), accounting for almost 80% of all motor vehicle traffic [4]. The healthcare sector contributes considerably to this overall traffic volume: the NHS in England, for example, moves 1.3 million staff, patients and visitor each day, accounting for about 5% of total road traffic emissions [5]. Much of this health-related road traffic (including getting to and from work) is due to single person car journeys, contributing to traffic congestion. Author Jane Holtz Kay aptly coined the phrase 'you're not stuck in a traffic jam, you are the jam' [6]. Road traffic not only causes carbon emissions but also affects human health directly by reducing air quality, causing road traffic crashes (no longer called 'accidents', which would imply that they are not preventable) and impairing access for people who are critically ill [7]. Estimates indicate that in cities such as Delhi, for example, more active travel could reduce heart attacks and strokes by 10–25% and diabetes by 6–17%, while lessening the impact through road traffic crashes by over 30% [8].

Reducing travel-related carbon emissions in healthcare

Health services can reduce travel and transport related carbon emissions in a number of areas (Figure 7.1).

Every healthcare facility is different, so analysing where emissions are greatest and the opportunities for reduction are most practical is a useful first step. An important part of this process is measuring personal and organisational carbon footprints using one of the available carbon footprint calculators (there is more information on these in Chapters 3 and 5).The following sections focus on models of care that help reduce carbon emissions while providing better services and saving money.

Reducing the need to travel

Travelling less has direct and immediate carbon benefits. To reduce the amount that patients and staff working in the health sector travel, we need to consider newer models of care and ways of communicating with each other.

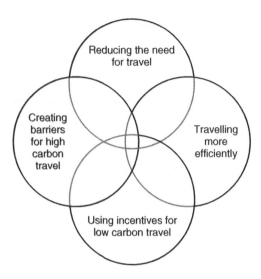

Figure 7.1 Options for reducing travel and transport-related carbon emissions.

Remote clinical care

Enabling staff to work remotely (for example, from their homes) can be an effective way of reducing travel. Apart from saving travelling time, transport costs and carbon emissions, working remotely can also increase job satisfaction and allow people to be more productive. Even greater gains can be achieved by empowering patients to manage acute and chronic medical themselves at home as and when appropriate. Telephone consultations can be an effective alternative to face-to-face consultations, and advances in information technology even allow remote computer access to local clinical servers from clinicians' homes. Telephone consultations and other forms of telemedicine have the potential to improve patient access and help manage clinical problems without the need for a face-to-face consultation, thereby reducing the need for travel. For example, the *Connected Work* programme introduced by *Partners Healthcare* used suburban satellite office space for teleworking and saved well over one million travel miles per year in 2010. Remote working may even save lives [9, 10], as also illustrated by Case study 7.1.

A related issue is the distance between home and work for the healthcare workforce. Where hospitals are near expensive residential locations, lower-paid hospital workers (perhaps those who prepare food or clean up) must often commute long distances. When they drive, they may drive the oldest, most polluting cars. Many hospitals provide nearby 'workforce housing',

Case study 7.1   Tele-radiology

In 1992, I returned from a radiology convention excited by a new technology I had seen. This technology allowed digitally acquired images, such as CT scans, to be transmitted over telephone lines and viewed remotely. Fortunately, I was working at a successful and forward thinking hospital that was eager to embrace new ideas and service improvements. In those days, if there was a CT scan to be read after hours, I would have to get up and dressed and drive the 20 minutes to the hospital. This would occur anywhere from one to six times a night. Obviously the idea of being able to perform that service in my pyjamas was enticing, saving the journeys and critical time in life and death situations. I managed to convince the hospital administration that entering this world of tele-radiology would be money well spent. One week after we had installed the system I was called about a patient with back pain and a known aortic aneurysm. Within five minutes of this call I had diagnosed that the aneurysm was leaking and instructed the radiographer to take the patient directly to the operating room. I also immediately contacted the surgeon and he operated as expeditiously as possible. He later told me that as he entered the abdomen the aneurysm burst in front of his eyes. The twenty minute drive I avoided may have saved that patient's life. My belief in this then very new technology was vindicated. Anything that can be digitised, seen on a scan, through a scope or on a slide can be reviewed by an expert anywhere in the world in a matter of minutes or hours. No longer will expert consultation require a pilgrimage, it only requires an Internet connection. Many interesting possibilities are emerging for high quality, high speed and low-carbon radiological care.

Reproduced with permission from Dr Kenneth J. Goodman, MD, FACR,
Chairman and Attending Physician, Department of Radiology,
St Francis Hospital, Roslyn, New York.

which reduces travel demand and encourages low-carbon transport [11]. Engaging with local housing authorities and property developers when planning new facilities can help to advance this goal.

Providing healthcare closer to home – or in the home

Providing health services closer to people's home can often avoid unnecessary patient travel, as long as facilities are easily accessible to patients, staff and visitors. Telemedicine – using telecommunication and information technology to provide clinical care remotely – can help reduce distance barriers and improve access to medical care. Transmitting patient data remotely is becoming increasingly common and can be life-saving. A recent systematic review shows that in patients with congestive heart failure, tele-monitoring in conjunction with nurse home visiting and specialist unit support can reduce the need for travel while maintaining quality of care and improving patients' quality of life [12]. Telemedicine systems can also improve the physical health of stroke patients, with both health practitioners and participants reporting high levels of satisfaction and acceptance [13]. And extrapolating travel data from a randomised controlled trial of general practitioner (GP)-led integrated follow up for people with cutaneous malignant melanoma, moving melanoma follow-up visits from hospital to primary care could potentially reduce annual carbon dioxide emissions in the United Kingdom by 1872 tonnes [14].

Teleworking and virtual meetings

Teleconferencing and videoconferencing are forms of virtual meetings among two or more participants that employ technology which is more sophisticated than a simple two-way phone connection. A simple *teleconference* can be an audio conference with one or both ends of the conference sharing a speaker phone. A *videoconference* can be conducted from a computer using software like *Skype* or, with much higher fidelity, through dedicated videoconferencing facilities. Both forms of conferencing can save a considerable amount of time and carbon, both in high and low-income countries [2]. Simple mobile phone applications are often all that is needed for supporting emergency assistance and facilitating long-distance consultations with healthcare workers, which is particularly relevant for creating better access to healthcare in remote areas [15]. Early results of the *Whole System Demonstrator Programme*, the largest randomised controlled trial of tele-health and tele-care in the world, involving 6191 patients and 238 GP practices in the United Kingdom, showed that, if used correctly, tele-health interventions can reduce emergency department visits by 15%, emergency admissions by 20% and elective admissions by 14% – and, even more strikingly, reduce mortality rates by 45% [16] (Case study 7.2).

Choosing local suppliers

Procurement is the biggest contributor to many health services' carbon footprints, contributing up to about 60% of carbon emissions within the UK

Case study 7.2   Benefits of teleconferencing

Staff at the NHS Derbyshire Community Health Services NHS Trust in the United Kingdom travel collectively around five million miles a year, leading to considerable expenses, wasting valuable travel time and causing carbon emissions [17]. Introducing teleconferencing led to 1200 teleconference calls with 4700 people taking part, saving more than 3000 hours of staff travel time and around 20 tons of carbon emissions – which also saved £100 000 (US$ 160 000) in the process. All that was needed was a fixed or mobile phone line. Up to 40 people regularly take part in teleconferences that last around 35 minutes, which are shorter and more focused than face-to-face meetings.

Case study 7.3   The Cornwall Food Programme [19]

Since 2001, the NHS in Cornwall (UK) has pioneered an innovative approach to buying and cooking food for its three flagship hospitals. The Cornwall Food Programme (CFP) offers nutritious food that is popular with patients, spending 40% of its budget within the local economy, and cutting 'food miles' travelled by delivery vehicles by 67%. This has been achieved within a daily food budget of £2.50 per person. For instance, a locally made fishcake has replaced the nationally procured alternative which for many patients was an unpopular food choice. The fishcake contains 40% locally caught fish combined with locally grown potatoes. Contracts for fruit and vegetables, meat, fresh milk, eggs and dried goods are now all awarded to Cornish companies.

National Health Service (NHS), part of which is due to transporting goods and services (there is more on this in Chapter 9) [18].

As Case study 7.3 illustrates, switching to local suppliers, particularly those which use carbon-efficient vehicles, is one of many practical steps that healthcare organisations can take to reduced travel-related emissions. Where travel cannot be avoided, using more efficient means of moving people and goods around is the next best option – and the topic of the next section.

Better ways to travel

When travel and transport cannot be avoided, there are often better ways of moving people and goods. Active travel in particular has many benefits.

Active travel: walking and cycling

Increasing the amount of 'active travel', such as walking and cycling, not only has carbon benefits. Where active travel leads to a shift away from a more sedentary lifestyle, people will also achieve co-benefits in terms of improving health and saving money [8]. The health and environmental benefits of active travel are considerable [20, 21]. Walking, for instance, reduces mortality from all causes, coronary heart disease, other cardiovascular disease, all cancers, respiratory disease and colorectal cancer [22]. A study published in the *Journal of the American Medical Association* in 1995 showed that men who maintained or improved their physical fitness were less likely to die from all causes or cardiovascular disease during the follow-up period than those who stayed unfit [23]. For cycling, studies show similar benefits. Impressively, a Danish study showed that the just under 7000 study participants who cycled to work had a 39% lower mortality rate after multivariate adjustment compared to those who did not [24]. But of course it is not only about mortality. Cyclists also have lower rates of sickness absence from work, so increasing cycling is likely to improve productivity [25].

Projections published in *The Lancet* in 2009 estimate that a combination of active travel and lower-emission motor vehicles could reduce the number of years of life lost from ischaemic heart disease in London by 10–19% and in Delhi by 11–25% [8]. Walking and cycling can have additional health and social benefits, which may not always be obvious or easily measurable. For example, these forms of active travel can help to improve the quality of life in areas that are exposed to heavy traffic, reduce social isolation, help fight obesity and generally help communities to grow together [26, 27]. This is particularly true for socially disadvantaged areas, where pedestrian child casualties are often higher than in more affluent neighbourhoods and where a shift from using the car to active travel may contribute to making roads safer [28]. Cycling has also been shown to have a positive effect on emotional health, levels of wellbeing, self-confidence and tolerance to stress, while improving sleep, reducing tiredness and problems with other physical symptoms [29].

Worldwide, motor vehicle collisions kill an estimated 1.2 million people every year (contributing to 2.2% of all deaths) and injure 50 million more [30]. In the United Kingdom there is evidence to suggest that child pedestrian injuries caused by cars are five times more common in deprived areas compared to the least deprived [31]. Findings from studies like these have led to major initiatives supported by numerous bodies (such as *Sustrans* in the United Kingdom) to encourage people to promote and take up active travel in preference to carbon-intensive, and ultimately unhealthy, ways of travel [32]. Although encouraging active travel should be a priority for any

Case study 7.4   Cycling family doctor

I started riding a bicycle as a student in London. Cycling as a GP in North Bristol (UK) is a lot less scary. It took me a while to take the plunge, put off by my colleagues' assertions that it was dangerous and impractical. Once in the saddle though, I was hooked. People assume that my motivations are virtuous – lowering my carbon footprint and keeping fit. These, however, are secondary to the sheer joy of cycling. I'm privileged to ride to work through ancient wooded parkland, spotting a kingfisher on occasions, but even during less rewarding urban cycling, something good seems to happen to my brain. I'm convinced that cycling makes me a more creative and cheerful doctor.

There are other effects: the burden of home visits is lightened by an opportunity for Vitamin D-boosting daylight and fresh air, and over-crowded head space clears on the ride home at the end of the day. It does also feel good to visibly lead a lifestyle that we promote, and I think there is a ripple effect. One patient, looking after his wife with Alzheimer's, has rejuvenated his bike to nip out to the local shops whilst her carers come. Only today I was hailed by a fellow cyclist who is a patient recovering from depression. We're lucky to have a Lifecycle UK locally, a charity helping people to develop confidence in their cycling skills (http://www.lifecycleuk.org.uk/).

So what are the downsides? I've been bitten by a bulldog ('only a puppy'), mistaken for the postman (red panniers) and castigated by the practice nurse for shaking up the emergency drugs box. Sound waterproofs are essential and reinforced tyres a good idea.

I'm wondering how many years my knees will cope with the hills, but an enthusiast tells me an electric bike could be the next step.

Dr Marion Steiner, General Practitioner, Bristol, UK (personal communication,
reproduced with permission)

organisation or employer, the health co-benefits are a particularly strong reason for the healthcare community to take an active lead. Clinicians and other people working in the health sector are ideally placed to lead by example. When clinicians take the leap to become car-free, this is not only healthier and low carbon but can also be a truly liberating experience, as illustrated in a personal account from a cycling family doctor in Bristol, UK (Case study 7.4).

Cycling can be a fun, healthy, cheap and clean alternative to car travel that is easy to take up and build into the daily routine [33]. Cycling can form an important part of clinical care, for example through the prescription of exercise in primary care [34]. However, we have to acknowledge the limits of active transport, in that patients or healthcare professionals will often be unable to walk or bike in, and visitors may be coming from far away and can be unfamiliar with the routes. By shifting to active forms of transport, the healthcare community has a great opportunity to set an example to the wider population.

Car pooling and car sharing

When car travel cannot be avoided, there is often scope for increasing the efficiency of car use in the health sector. Car pooling is an arrangement whereby more than one person occupies the same vehicle, often sharing cost and taking turns as the driver. Car pooling not only reduces the stress of driving a car – it also saves on fuel, reduces carbon emissions as well as traffic congestion, and it eases the need for car parking spaces [35]. A good place to start to incentivise multiple occupancy vehicle (MOV) travel is to provide free parking spaces for them.

Car sharing is a form of car rental where people hire cars for short periods of time, often by the hour. The cars may be rented by a commercial business, or users may get together and form a company or cooperative themselves. Car sharing has become popular in hundreds of cities worldwide. If people decide to take part in a car-sharing scheme, they can save money by avoiding the costs and responsibilities of car ownership while still having access to cars, and they are more likely to use active transport as an alternative when possible [36]. Where car sharing and car pooling initiatives improve access and reliability, they may also lead to greater staff satisfaction in addition to carbon savings [37, 38]. Because petroleum products are intrinsic to modern healthcare, and shifts in petroleum supply can affect healthcare prices, saving fuel not only reduces carbon emissions but also helps to increase resilience [39].

Fuel efficient vehicles

It is not only patient, staff and visitor travel that contribute to the health sector's travel emissions. Many health services also have their own or leased fleets of vehicles, such as ambulances, mini-buses or other transport vehicles. Where health systems use their collective buying power, there is scope to specify particularly low-carbon vehicles when leasing or buying new vehicles [38]. For example, *Partners HealthCare* in Boston, USA, has specified the use of ultra-low-sulfur diesel in its construction contracts. Health services

---

Case study 7.5 'Green Ambulances' in Sweden [41]

In 2001, one of Stockholm's leading ambulance operators, AISAB, aimed to create a 'green ambulance service' [41]. Its key criteria included that ambulance engines run on renewable fuels, that all materials in the ambulance are sourced with environmental considerations in mind and that all ambulance drivers follow a driving style that makes more efficient use of fuel – not by driving slower but by driving smarter through planning ahead. Results showed that a change in driving practice (which has now become mandatory for all ambulance operators in Stockholm) led to an average 3–4% lower fuel consumption (with a possible maximum of 10%), 50% fewer insurance claims and lower wear of tyres and brakes. Although drivers were sceptical initially, there was no increased risk to patients – and the drivers even went into competition on who used the least fuel.

---

can also demand certain carbon emission criteria from other services, such as taxi companies. Hybrid engines using two or more power sources to move vehicles are more fuel efficient than traditional combustion engines through their built-in electric battery. Trends suggest that all major car makers will be promoting smaller, high efficiency vehicles vigorously in the next few years [40]. A good example of how vehicles can be used more efficiently comes from Sweden (Case study 7.5) [41].

Incentivising active travel

For those who normally drive, switching to active travel or public transport requires a major change in behaviour. Creating the right incentives and barriers can facilitate such change.

Car parking

Car parking spaces are expensive to build and take up considerable space. They also incur regular costs for maintenance, security, lighting and cleaning – all resources that could be better used for patient care [38]. Car parking control is critical for changing travel behaviour and choice of transport mode. When car parking spaces are cheap or free, they largely subsidise those who travel by car (often those people with higher incomes within an organisation) with no such comparable subsidy to those who choose or have to use other modes of transport.

If you are involved in planning, constructing or managing car parking facilities, consider reducing the number of free or subsidised car parking spaces to encourage active and other alternative ways of travelling. Also think about rewarding multiple occupancy vehicles (MOVs) and lower emission transport, especially bicycles and hybrid cars. As this is likely to cause opposition, it is usually best to plan, pilot and introduce alternative travel arrangements before reducing the availability of car parking spaces, so that staff and patients can still travel safely and effectively. This process needs to be transparent and show that there is a priority list of who is entitled to park a vehicle on site and that there are parking rules which will be enforced. There will often be scope to reduce the number of parking space users to a relatively small number by establishing a pool of fleet vehicles. This can help with making non-car travel a more attractive option by creating a stronger incentive [42].

Mileage allowances for business travel and training

Business travel and travel for staff training, professional development and conferences is a significant part of health sector travel (Chapter 11). Wherever possible, meetings, conferences and training days should take place in locations that are close to the whereabouts of the participants [38]. Preferred venues should also be easily accessible by active and public transport. Modern information technology allows for new ways of passing on information that make is less necessary to attend events in person. Options include podcasting, webinars, meeting webcasting and teleconferencing, which can all be convenient and cost effective while carrying a considerably lower carbon footprint (Chapter 11). Air travel should only be used in exceptional cases. To encourage active travel, health services may consider reimbursing lower-carbon vehicles at higher rates than those with a larger engine size. Ideally, they should pay the maximum rates for people who use lower carbon options such as public transport or cycling [38].

Institutional travel plans

Transport needs and arrangements for providing healthcare will vary, depending on the needs of the population and available facilities in a particular area. Whatever the setting, a sensible first step is to review the travel needs for staff, patients and visitors and develop an 'institutional travel plan' promoting and encouraging sustainable transport, particularly active travel. It is good practice to make such plans public through adverts and within staff induction packs [37, 38] (Case study 7.6.) Where travel plans lead to financial savings, these can be ploughed back into providing clinical care.

Case study 7.6   Creating an institutional travel plan

Addenbrookes Hospital in Cambridge, UK, provides a good example of how creating a travel plan that was initially launched in 1993 has helped patients, visitors and staff travel to and from their campus more effectively. Having been presented with the Cambridgeshire and Peterborough Travel Plan Excellence Award in 2005, the hospital tries hard to reduce the demand for car travel by promoting and supporting alternative modes of travel [43]. These include walking to the campus, providing 60 buses an hour through its own shuttle service, using five park-and-ride sites and making available 1300 cycle parking spaces on site. Addenbrooke's travel plan successfully managed to reduce the number of staff travelling to their site by single occupancy car travel from 50% in 2000 to 34% in 2007, and the number of patients and visitors who travel by car decreased from 92% in 2002 to 85% in 2007.

So what are the areas that such travel plans should cover, and how can travel plans be implemented and monitored?

Monitoring and measuring

Understanding an organisation's travel needs and travel-related emissions means calculating baseline emissions and the resulting carbon footprint. Various tools have been developed that allow capturing travel-related data. The Carbon Trust and the UK Royal College of General Practitioners, for example, have produced good introductions to carbon footprinting [44, 45].

Public transport

Using public transport instead of cars not only contributes to lowering carbon emissions, but also forms an important component of active travel in that people who use public transport get more exercise than those who drive a car [46]. To make best use of public transport, the location of healthcare facilities is crucial. For example, healthcare premises in city centres usually have good transport links, whereas hospitals built on a ring road encourage car use. Liaising with a local bus company may help ensure adequate bus access, and local councils may be prepared to fund extra services at off-peak times.

Case study 7.7   Petrol-free community team [50]

A community healthcare team in Bristol has gone 'petrol free' by adding an electric car to its fleet of four electric bicycles as part of a wider initiative to reduce its travel-related carbon footprint. Changing from cars to bicycles means that members of the team avoid traffic jams in Bristol's busy traffic, thereby often getting to clients faster and feeling healthier from walking and cycling – both physically and mentally.

Behaviour change

Travel habits are often entrenched, and incentives are needed to catalyse behavioural change (Case study 7.7). The *Cycle to Work Scheme* in the United Kingdom (www.bike2workscheme.co.uk), for instance, allows organisations to offer their employees a 'tax free' bicycle as part of their employment package [47]. It should be as easy as possible for people to travel actively to healthcare premises. Good evidence exists that people are in favour of establishing transport strategies and policies that encourage and support active travel such as cycling and walking as well as public transport, even if this disadvantages drivers of private cars [48, 49]. Encouraging personalised travel plans and working with people at transition times, such as starting new job or moving house, are often the best times to bring about a change in habit [42].

In many major cities, cycling is on the increase. New York has started to build bike lanes, cities like Montreal or London have created public bike schemes, while Amsterdam and Beijing have long traditions of being bike-friendly. The reasons for this increase in cycling are multifaceted, but perhaps the messages about the health benefits are getting through. There is no doubt that increasing numbers of cyclists in cities change their 'feel' and gives aide to the concept of 'safety in numbers' – the more pedestrians and/or cyclists the safer active travel becomes.

Infrastructure for active travel

Healthcare organisations that wish to nurture active travel need to provide basic infrastructure, such as lockers, rooms for drying clothes, showers, changing rooms, secure covered storage for bicycles and the 'bike to work schemes' mentioned earlier. Healthcare providers also play an important role in pushing for better infrastructure outside their facilities', borders such as better pavements (sidewalks) and bike trails. Linking up with local transport partners can facilitate this process enormously.

Moving into action!

Considering newer and better models of care is an effective way to make transport and travel in the health sector more sustainable. The potential health benefits from active travel and reducing travel-related emissions are substantial. And probably even more important is the role that healthcare organisations can take through *leadership* and *lobbying*. Health systems around the world have a great opportunity to be shining examples. They are powerful forces (for example, the UK NHS is one of the largest employers in the world, next to the Indian railways and the Chinese People's Liberation Army), so it has a great opportunity, and a duty, to use that power to best effect by driving local authorities, other strategic partners and even governments to adopt more sustainable (and active travel friendly) policies and strategies. Clinicians have great opportunities for reducing patient-related travel – by using telephone consultations instead of face-to-face contacts whenever possible, and by talking to their patients about using active travel where suitable.

In this chapter we have outlined the environmental as well as health benefits from moving people and goods in the health sector better – and, more importantly, less. Avoiding carbon-intensive travel can often instantly save substantial amounts of money. And making use of new technologies such as telemedicine not only saves time, money and carbon, but can also lead to better patient care.

So using more sustainable transport and implementing sustainable transport policies makes sense from many viewpoints. But transport is only one part of the story and the next chapter looks at where much travel starts and ends: near buildings and spaces.

Key actions for implementing institutional travel plans

If your healthcare organisation does not have an institutional travel plan, the following list of key tasks may help with planning and implementation. Because of their time, motion and cost benefits they may also provide key arguments with administrators [38]:

- *Use active travel*: Travel by bike, on foot or with public transport as often as you can. Make it a point to avoid flying as much as possible. Always lead by example.
- *Get involved*: Get involved in your organisation's travel plan and actively support sustainability related travel initiatives.
- *Enable good leadership*: Unless it is you, check out who is responsible for travel planning in your organisation and discuss what they

are doing to encourage active travel. Unless you have a steering group, suggest that your organisation creates one with support and leadership at senior level. All healthcare providers should have a board approved active travel plan as part of an overall sustainable development management plan.

- *Communicate your plan*: Publicise, market and campaign for your organisation's new approach to travelling for all staff, patients and visitors through any of your communications, such as websites, stationery, information leaflets, and posters.
- *Set targets*: Set targets for reducing the number of single occupancy car journeys to your healthcare site and ensure this is line with any national, regional and local sustainable development action plans.
- *Measure carbon emissions*: Make sure that your organisation has structures in place to monitor transport-related carbon emissions, so that these can be measured. Routinely monitor and review the need for staff and patient travel, and look for opportunities to reduce these. Perform full life cycle analyses that include goods and services (there is more on this in Chapter 3).
- *Promote active and alternative travel*: Encourage people to travel more sustainably to and from your site – cycling, walking, car sharing/pooling and using public transport such as buses or trains are good examples. Try to negotiate discounts for staff and patients with local public transport providers.
- *Reduce travel*: Where possible, reduce the number of journeys undertaken for work by offering and promoting alternatives such as web, video and teleconferencing.
- *Favour sustainable travel*: Introduce a flat rate for business mileage, regardless of the mode of transport – preferably with higher rates for active transport and vehicles that have higher energy efficiency ratings.
- *Location of facilities*: Provide care closer to home where possible.
- *Create a supportive infrastructure*: Provide lockers, showers, secure bike storage, better route lighting, appropriate signing and other facilities that encourage and remove barriers for active travel.
- *Promote the business case for active travel*: Make people aware of the co-benefits of active travel, which include improved physical fitness, increased mental wellbeing, reduced sickness absence staff turnover – all of which may also have direct financial benefits.
- *Collaborate*: Work together with staff, the local community, other businesses and transport providers to produce a travel plan that is custom-made for your area. Promote sharing facilities and transport

with other individuals and local organisations to increase the opportunities for alternatives to car use.
• *Advocate*: Advocate for progressive transport strategies.

References

1. NHS Sustainable Development Unit (2012) Sustainability in the NHS: Health Check 2012 [Internet]. http://www.sdu.nhs.uk/healthcheck2012 [accessed 21 February 2012].
2. WHO – Health in the Green Economy [Internet]. http://www.who.int/hia/green_economy/en/index.html [accessed 26 October 2011].
3. Sidell, M., Jones, L., Katz, J. and Peberdy, A. (2003) *Debates and Dilemmas in Promoting Health. A Reader*. Open University/Palgrave Macmillan, UK.
4. Department for Transport – Road traffic statistics [Internet]. http://www.dft.gov.uk/pgr/statistics/datatablespublications/roads/traffic/index.html [accessed 17 August 2011].
5. NHS Confederation (2007) Taking the temperature: Towards an NHS response to global warming [Internet]. http://www.nhsconfed.org/Publications/Documents/Taking%20the%20temperature.pdf [accessed 15 July 2011].
6. Kay, J. (1997) *Asphalt nation: how the automobile took over America, and how we can take it back*. Crown Publishers, New York.
7. Davis, R.M. (2001) BMJ bans 'accidents'. *British Medical Journal*, **322**, 1320–1321.
8. Woodcock, J., Edwards, P., Tonne, C. *et al.* (2009) Public health benefits of strategies to reduce greenhouse-gas emissions: urban land transport. *Lancet*, **374** (9705), 1930–1943.
9. Bunn, F., Byrne, G. and Kendall, S. (2004) Telephone consultation and triage: effects on health care use and patient satisfaction. *Cochrane Database of Systematic Reviews*, (4):CD004180.
10. Beaver, K., Tysver-Robinson, D., Campbell, M. *et al.* (2009) Comparing hospital and telephone follow-up after treatment for breast cancer: randomised equivalence trial. *British Medical Journal*, **338**, a3147.
11. Heatherwood and Wexham Park Hospitals – Staff Benefits [Internet]. http://www.heatherwoodandwexham.nhs.uk/work/staff-benefits-frequently-asked-questions [accessed 26 November 2011].
12. Clarke, M., Shah, A. and Sharma, U. (2010) Systematic review of studies on telemonitoring of patients with congestive heart failure: a meta-analysis. *Journal of Telemedicine and Telecare*, **17**, 7–14.
13. Johansson, T. and Wild, C. (2010) Telerehabilitation in stroke care – a systematic review. *Journal of Telemedicine and Telecare*, **17**, 1–6.
14. Murchie, P. (2007) Environmental impact of GP-led melanoma follow up. *British Journal of General Practice*, **57** (543), 837–538.
15. Wooton, R., Patil, N., Scott, R. and Ho, K. (2009) *Telehealth in the Developing World*. The Royal Society of Medicine Ltd Press, London.

16. UK Department of Health (2011) Whole system demonstrator programme. Headline findings(December 2011) [Internet]. http://www.dh.gov.uk/en/Pub licationsandstatistics/Publications/PublicationsPolicyAndGuidance/DH_131684 [accessed 24 February 2012].

17. NHS Sustainable Development Unit – Case Study: Teleconferencing [Internet]. http://www.sdu.nhs.uk/documents/case_study/Teleconferencing.pdf [accessed 24 October 2011].

18. NHS Sustainable Development Unit (2009) NHS England Carbon Emissions Carbon Footprinting Report (September 2008; updated August 2009) [Internet]. http://www.sdu.nhs.uk/documents/publications/1263313924_jgyW_nhs _england_carbon_emissions_carbon_footprinting_r.pdf [accessed 12 September 2011].

19. Cornwall Food Programme website (Home) [Internet]. http://www.cornwallfood programme.co.uk/ [accessed 21 February 2012].

20. Oja, P., Titze, S., Bauman, A., de Geus, B. *et al.* (2011) Health benefits of cycling: a systematic review. *Scandinavian Journal of Medicine & Science in Sports*, **21**, 496–509.

21. de Nazelle, A., Nieuwenhuijsen, M.J., Antó, J.M. *et al.* (2011) Improving health through policies that promote active travel: a review of evidence to support integrated health impact assessment. *Environment International*, **37** (4), 766–777.

22. Davey Smith, G., Shipley, M.J., Batty, G.D., Morris, J.N. and Marmot, M. (2000) Physical activity and cause-specific mortality in the Whitehall study. *Public Health*, **114** (5), 308–315.

23. Blair, S.N., Kohl, III, H.W., Barlow, C.E., Paffenbarger, R.S. Jr, Gibbons, L.W. and Macera, C.A. (1995) Changes in physical fitness and all-cause mortality. *A prospective study of healthy and unhealthy men. Journal of the American Medical Association*, **273** (14), 1093–1098.

24. Andersen, L.B., Schnohr, P., Schroll, M. and Hein, H.O. (2000) All-cause mortality associated with physical activity during leisure time, work, sports, and cycling to work. *Archives of Internal Medicine*, **160** (11), 1621–1628.

25. TNO (2009) Reduced sickness absence in regular commuter cyclists can save employers 27 million euros [Internet]. http://www.vcl.li/bilder/518.pdf [accessed 22 October 2011].

26. UK Department of Health (2004) At least five a week: Evidence on the impact of physical activity and its relationship to health [Internet]. http:// www.dh.gov.uk/en/Publicationsandstatistics/Publications/PublicationsPolicy AndGuidance/DH_4080994 [accessed 18 August 2012].

27. The British Medical Association – Road transport and health [Internet]. http://bma.org.uk/search?query=Road%20transport%20and%20health [access ed 23 October 2011].

28. Audit Commission (2007) Better safe than sorry [Internet]. http://www.audit-commission.gov.uk/nationalstudies/childrenyoungpeople/Pages/bettersafethan sorry.aspx [accessed 23 October 2011].

29. Boyd, H., Hillman, M., Nevill, A., Pearce, L.P. and Tuxworth, B. Health related effects of regular cycling on a sample of previous non-exercisers. CTC and Bike For Your Life Project (1998) [Internet]. http://webarchive.nationalarchives.gov.uk/

+/http://www.dft.gov.uk/pgr/roads/tpm/tal/cyclefacilities/cyclingforbetterhealth [accessed 23 October 2011].

30. WHO (2004) World report on road traffic injury prevention [Internet]. [cited 2011 Oct 23]. Available from: http://www.who.int/violence_injury_prevention/ publications/road_traffic/world_report/en/index.html [accessed 23 October 2011].

31. UK Department of Health (2003) Tackling health inequalities: A Programme for Action [Internet]. http://www.dh.gov.uk/en/Publicationsandstatistics/ Publications/PublicationsPolicyAndGuidance/DH_4008268 [accessed 18 August 2011].

32. Sustrans – Active commuting and travel plans: help and advice [Internet]. http://www.sustrans.org.uk/what-we-do/active-travel/active-travel-information-resources/active-commuting-and-travel-plans-help-and-advice [accessed 17 August 2011].

33. Shephard, R.J. (1992) A critical analysis of work-site fitness programs and their postulated economic benefits. *Medicine and Science in Sports and Exercise*, **24** (3), 354–370.

34. Khan, K.M., Weiler, R. and Blair, S.N. (2011) Prescribing exercise in primary care. *British Medical Journal*, **343**, d4141.

35. Zipcar – Car sharing, an alternative to car rental and car ownership [Internet].http://www.zipcar.com/ [accessed 21 February 2012].

36. Shaheen, S.A., Cohen, A.P. and Chung, M.S. (2009) North American Carsharing. *Transportation Research Record: Journal of the Transportation Research Board*, **2110** (1), 35–44.

37. NHS Sustainable Development Unit (2009) *Saving Carbon*, Improving Health: Carbon Reduction Strategy for England. NHS Sustainable Development Unit, Cambridge.

38. NHS Sustainable Development Unit – NHS Carbon Reduction Strategy: Extended chapters [Internet]. http://www.sdu.nhs.uk/publications-resources/46/NHS-Carbon-Reduction-Strategy--Extended-chapters/ [accessed 18 August 2011].

39. Hess, J., Bednarz, D., Bae, J. and Pierce, J. (2011) Petroleum and Health Care: Evaluating and Managing Health Care's Vulnerability to Petroleum Supply Shifts. *American Journal of Public Health*, **101**, 1568–1579.

40. Plunkett Research Ltd – Automobiles trucks market research: trends [Internet]. http://www.plunkettresearch.com/Automobiles%20trucks%20market%20resear ch/industry%20overview [accessed 18 August 2011].

41. AISAB (2010) The Green Ambulance [Internet]. http://sustainablehealthcare.files. wordpress.com/2010/05/eco-driving-green-ambulance.pdf [accessed 19 August 2011].

42. Verplanken, B. (2004) Habits and implementation intentions. In: J. Kerr, R. Weitkunat and M. Moretti (eds) *The ABC of Behavior Change: A Guide to Successful Disease Prevention and Health Promotion*, pp. 99–109. Elsevier Science, Oxford.

43. Addenbrooke's Hospital (2005) Yet another success for hospital's travel plan! [Internet]. http://www.addenbrookes.org.uk/news/news2005/sep/travel_award_ 09.09.05.html [accessed 19 August 2011].

44. Carbon Trust – Footprint measurement [Internet]. http://www.carbontrust.co.
    uk/cut-carbon-reduce-costs/calculate/footprint-calculator/pages/footprinting-
    tools.aspx [accessed 18 August 2011].
45. Royal College of General Practitioners – Carbon footprint calculator [Internet].
    http://www.rcgp.org.uk/professional_development/carbon_footprint_calculator
    .aspx [accessed 22 October 2011].
46. Besser, L.M. and Dannenberg, A.L. (2005) Walking to public transit: steps to help
    meet physical activity recommendations. *American Journal of Preventive Medicine*,
    29 (4), 273–280.
47. Cycle Solutions – The Cycle to Work Scheme [Internet]. http://www.cyclesolu
    tions.co.uk/?gclid=CM_W9Y-32KoCFRJc4QodI0dF7w [accessed 18 August
    2011].
48. UK Department for Transport (2011) 2010 British Social Attitudes Survey: Atti-
    tudes to transport [Internet]. http://www.dft.gov.uk/publications/2010-british-
    social-attitudes-survey-attitudes-to-transport [accessed 23 October 2011].
49. Sustrans – Travel Behaviour Research Baseline Service [Internet]. http://www.
    sustrans.org.uk/search-results?search=Travel+Behaviour+Research+Baseline+
    Survey [accessed 18 August 2011].
50. Avon and Wiltshire Mental Health Partnership NHS Trust (AWP) – Bristol
    community healthcare team go petrol free [Internet]. http://www.awp.nhs.uk/tem
    plates/page_3258.aspx [accessed 21 February 2012].

Chapter 8 **Healthy buildings, healthy spaces**

In this chapter

- Looking at the impacts of buildings and spaces in healthcare
- Creating more sustainable buildings and spaces
- Achieving better energy efficiency
- The effect of the natural environment on health

The building in healthcare

In an essay on the history of architecture and health, Edwin Heathcote captures the way in which healthcare buildings have evolved from antiquity to modern times: 'Over its long, rich and varied history, the architecture of health has been a monument to the gods, a monument to God, and, ultimately, a monument to science. What it has rarely been is a monument to mankind' [1]. From a practical perspective, healthcare buildings are more than monuments, of course: they are living, breathing buildings with an important job to do. They are where people are born and die, where illness is discovered and cured. They are complex spaces in which people's existential and physical needs intersect. And it has been shown that the way in which these spaces are designed has an effect on the wellbeing and experience of patients and staff [2].

The earliest evidence of healthcare buildings is of temples in Ancient Egypt and Greece. Priest-physicians used these temples for the care of the sick, tending to their physical and spiritual needs. The Roman writer Vitruvius (born 80 BC) wrote about the best positioning of temples to promote health. The Romans also brought the healthcare building into the network of civic architecture, with a decree in AD 325 that all cities have a hospital [1]. In the grim parts of the Victorian metropolis, however, workhouse infirmaries, the

Sustainable Healthcare, First Edition. Knut Schroeder, Trevor Thompson, Kathleen Frith and David Pencheon.
© 2013 John Wiley & Sons, Ltd. Published 2013 by John Wiley & Sons, Ltd.

only hospitals that the poorest people had access to, were places from which people rarely returned. Poor hygiene and overcrowded conditions meant infections and disease were rife [3].

Increased medical knowledge led to developments in the architecture of healthcare buildings. Understanding the spread of disease changed the way in which hospitals were designed, with the circulation of fresh air and natural light being among the specified design characteristics of a more hygienic hospital. The nineteenth century ideals of Florence Nightingale of 'provisions for adequate ventilation, odour reduction in painted and papered rooms, and windows that offered natural light and pleasant views' remain central to the design of sustainable healthcare buildings today [4].

With advances in technology in the twentieth and twenty-first centuries, healthcare buildings needed to house increasing amounts medical equipment. This often resulted in environments which were more functional than aesthetic, 'more machine than monument'. In response to this 'mechanisation', the notion of *Evidence-Based Design (EBD)* emerged. EBD is 'the process of basing decisions about the built environment on credible research to achieve the best possible outcomes' [5]. This now well-established architectural approach uses the patient experience as the central design focus for healthcare buildings; for instance, lowering stress by giving patients control over lighting and temperature in their immediate environment [6, 7].

Today, we have over 17 000 hospitals on the planet [8]. But the traditional way in which health services use buildings is changing. For instance, patients with mental health conditions are increasingly being treated in the community rather than in institutions [9]. Frail and dependent people are more and more being cared for at home, and specialist nurses manage chronic diseases in the community rather than in hospitals [10, 11]. In patients with heart failure who were admitted to selected hospitals in the United States, the mean length of hospital stay decreased by 28%, from 8.8 to 6.3 days, between 1993 and 2006 [12]. Childbirth provides another example: although babies are still largely delivered in hospital, women who have an uncomplicated delivery can now expect to be discharged within hours [13]. With services being re-located in the community, there is an increasing need for suitably equipped primary care centres. This often involves extending and retrofitting existing buildings. Although the time spent by patients within designated healthcare buildings may reduce, their role in facilitating high quality healthcare continues to be an important one.

Building for healing

Healthcare buildings, however thoughtfully built, do not provide care. The role of the building is a supportive one; a catalyst and container for the work of the staff and the recovery of the patients within it. In this context, the supportive qualities of the building are enhanced when the space is planned and designed to be sustainable. Edward Wilson's *biophilia hypothesis* suggests that human beings and other living systems share an instinctive bond, and that we humans feel better in a natural environment [14–16]. A sustainable building, built with awareness of its natural environment, such as in the use of natural materials (wood, stone, natural textiles), access to daylight and outside space, reconnects its staff and patients to the natural environment [17]. In doing so, the building uses nature to meet important psychological and emotional, as well as physical, needs [18]. For instance, patients recovering from surgery in rooms with an outdoor view have been shown to suffer fewer complications, use less pain medication and recover more quickly than those whose view was restricted to a brick wall [19]. The use natural motifs is part of the design in two United Kingdom hospitals, as described in case studies later in this chapter.

Incorporating domestic or 'home-like' qualities is another important element for the creation of a healing environment [20]. Giving attention to interior design aspects, such as colour, lighting and artwork, has been shown to help improve the experience for patients and their families. Space for family to stay is also a consideration (Case study 8.1). A pull-down bed in a children's hospital for a parent to stay alongside their sick child [21], or a double bed in a birth centre to allow a father to stay with his partner and newborn baby are small augmentations that can radically alter the patient experience.

Being able to personalise space and to manage their own surroundings in terms of light and noise has impacted positively on patients' sense of wellbeing [2]. If this need for control is met and patients feel comfortable, patients may become more flexible and forgiving of any other shortcomings relating to their environment. For example, in a post-occupancy evaluation

---

Case study 8.1   Evelina Children's Hospital

The Evelina Children's hospital at Guy's and St Thomas's, London, is described as 'a hospital that doesn't feel like a hospital'. Sunlight, fresh air ventilation and a four-storey conservatory that houses a gallery, performance space and cafe, create an uninstitutional space. Each of the seven floors is themed to the natural world, with visual symbols and themed artwork on the walls to help people find their way around. Staff and patients were consulted on the layout, design and colour schemes, and to ensure that the functional needs of the hospital were met by the new design.

Case study 8.2 Maggie's Centres

Maggie's Centres in the United Kingdom aim to empower people to live with, through and beyond cancer by bringing together professional help, communities of support and building design to create exceptional centres for cancer care. These centres are for anyone affected by cancer. They offer support for people during diagnosis, treatment, recurrence, at the end of life or in bereavement, or dealing with issues of survivorship. The kitchen table is at the heart of each centre, and the buildings' intimate scale and domestic interiors aim to put people at ease from the moment they walk through the door. The thoughtfully designed centres are built to a brief based upon the experience of someone living with cancer. They offer a 'fluid' space in which people can move between areas of community, such as the kitchen, and places that allow quiet contemplation as required. Their informal character facilitates the work of professional staff to support the emotional, practical and social needs of people living with cancer.

---

of Maggie's Dundee Centre, occasionally high noise levels were met with a high degree of forgiveness, which was attributed to the centre's light, warmth and interior design (Case study 8.2) [22, 23].

The preferred elements for a healthcare environment mostly relate to the natural world, such as letting in natural light or looking out onto green space. This common theme suggests a need for patients to connect with the world beyond the healthcare building. A sustainable approach to healthcare buildings, therefore, ensures the best outcome for society in the long term while at the same time responding to the needs of the people who use these buildings (Case studies 8.1 and 8.3).

Green spaces and health

Healthcare buildings provide a space in which patients and staff can feel safe from the elements. Yet the natural environment around healthcare buildings also contributes to the quality of life of patients, staff and visitors [25]. Because of this important interconnection between buildings and their surroundings, integrating green spaces into the planning of the building is essential. A considerable body of evidence supports the claim that direct contact with nature (in addition to looking at nature as described earlier) directly promotes health as well as physical and psychological wellbeing [18]. The natural environment is therefore a valuable resource for healthcare

Case study 8.3   Glasgow Homoeopathic Hospital

The Glasgow Homoeopathic Hospital (GHH) recognised that the physical environment affects people's health, particularly if they are unwell or vulnerable. To offer patients and staff a more healing environment, the GHH set out to create a place of beauty and healing. A design team involving clinicians, administrators, architects and artists managed to create an award-winning functional hospital of particular beauty that complies with NHS guidelines for quality standards, operating efficiency and cost. Part of this hospital's vision was to re-humanise care using a model that could be replicated in other settings.

The building uses an L-shaped structure that surrounds a carefully landscaped garden, which aims to break up the sense of institutional regularity but also allows the natural world to become part of the healing environment. Natural, recyclable and environmentally friendly materials such as wooden and linoleum floors, recyclable zinc for the roof and cane or non-allergenic leather furniture all help to create an 'organic' feel. Further details and a virtual tour of the premises are available at the GHH website [24].

Case study 8.4   Green and blue gyms

'Green Gym' programmes involve people in activities that improve the natural environment. In a national evaluation in the United Kingdom, taking part in such schemes led not only to mental health benefits in terms of boosts in self-esteem but also to increased confidence in almost 100% of participants through learning new skills and completing different tasks [28]. In a similar way, the *Blue Gym Campaign* supports different activities aiming to get more people physically active in and around coastal and inland waters [29, 30].

(Case study 8.4). Evidence suggests that safe green spaces may even be as effective as prescription drugs [26, 27].

Other health benefits of the natural environment include opportunities for increasing social contacts or assisting patient recovery after medical procedures such as surgery [31]. According to a systematic review published in 2011, 68% of included papers found an association between the lack of green space and obesity-related health indicators, although findings were inconsistent and mixed across studies [32]. People with easy access to safe

---

Case study 8.5 'Open' psychotherapy and counselling

Providing healthcare out in the open is an approach taken by the Tuke Centre in York, UK, for example. This organisation has gone as far as to run regular psychotherapy and counselling sessions during eight mile walks (reassuringly at a gentle pace), which give people time and space to think and talk about work-related mental health issues [36].

---

green spaces are more likely to exercise more and be less obese [33]. A study performed in The Netherlands showed that 15 out of 24 major physical diseases (including conditions such as coronary heart disease, diabetes, migraine and asthma) were lower among those people living closer to green spaces, which provided oases of improved health [34]. Contact with nature in the workplace may also reduce stress. Workers who could view trees and flowers have been shown to feel less stressed and more satisfied with their jobs than those who could only see built environments from their windows [35]. Protecting and integrating nature is, therefore, not only crucial from an environmental point of view (Chapters 1 and 2), but can also help reduce the burden of many mental and physical diseases (Case study 8.5).

Healthcare estate: carbon and resource impacts

Health systems around the globe make use of large estates. The UK National Health Service (NHS), for example, has the largest property portfolio in Europe, with an estate that comprises 25 million m^2 of occupied floor area at a value of £36 billion (US$ 58 billion) for buildings and equipment [37]. Consequently, the ecological footprint from healthcare buildings is substantial, particularly in high-income countries. In England alone, buildings used by the NHS use up over £410 million (US$ 658 million) worth of energy every year, emitting an estimated 3.7 million tonnes of carbon dioxide in the process (this is roughly the equivalent to one person flying economy class from London to Hong Kong and back one million times) [38, 39]. Such energy use contributed to about 22% of the NHS's carbon footprint between 1992 and 2004 in terms of relative carbon emissions [38]. This is not surprising, as the day-to-day running of hospitals, general practices and other healthcare facilities involves many energy-dependent processes (Figure 8.1).

Where fossil fuels heat or power buildings, high carbon emissions often go hand in hand with high fuel costs. Because of rising prices and the threat of *peak oil* (Chapter 1) [40], some health services already suffer fuel shortages, and many others are at risk of facing supply problems in the

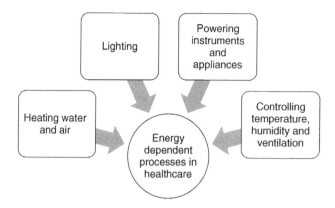

Figure 8.1 Examples of energy dependent activities in healthcare buildings.

future. As a result, switching to less carbon intensive forms of energy and using buildings and energy more efficiently make both environmental and financial sense. In addition, more efficient and sustainable buildings help increase the resilience of healthcare providers to predicted fluctuations in price and supply (Chapter 3). And financial savings from using new and better ways of managing energy can be substantial: in the United Kingdom, for example, projected energy efficiency savings could save the NHS an estimated £65 million (US$ 104 million) a year [41].

But there is also pressure from the top. Because of emerging national and international regulations and legislation, various bodies around the world have set standards that guide healthcare and other sectors towards best practice in sustainable design, construction and the running of buildings, including efficient energy use. These bodies include, for example:

- US Green Building Council: *Green Leadership in Energy and Environmental Design, LEED* [42].
- UK Building Research Establishment, BRE: The *Building Research Establishment's Environmental Assessment Method (BREEAM)* [43].
- Green Building Council, Australia: *Green Star – Healthcare* [44].
- Abu Dhabi Urban Planning Council, United Arab Emirates: *Estidama* [45].

These organisations use methods that are among the most comprehensive and widely recognised measures of buildings' environmental performance. Direct and lifetime carbon emissions are among their main benchmarks and aim to stimulate health service providers and other organisations to achieve the highest ratings with the lowest possible carbon impact. In the United States, an *Environmental Impact Calculator* is available from *Practice Greenhealth* [46]. This fairly simple analytical tool makes the connection between the quantity of energy being consumed, the profile of the energy source and potential health and economic outcomes.

Barriers to making buildings more sustainable

The principles of sustainable building design are similar for new builds and retrofits of existing buildings. Healthcare buildings are often designed in a way that locks their users into habits and models of care. Where such models of care are unsustainable or patient needs have changed, modifying poorly designed and inflexible structures can be difficult – and costly. Although retrofitting existing buildings and using sustainable practices for new building projects has multiple advantages because of *virtuous cycles* (Chapter 3), leading to benefits for the environment, the local community and the economy, myths about sustainable building are still widespread (Figure 8.2) [7, 47].

In the following sections we point out important design and other issues that are relevant for both new builds and retrofit projects of established buildings – with the latter being a more immediate and important area.

"Green" building is a passing fad	• no - green building principles have been used for centuries - but we have forgotten many of them
"Green" materials are not available	• no - recycled and environmenttally friendly materials are often widely available, and can be much cheaper
"Green" building is easy - it's only common sense	• no - green building is a holistic concept that requires careful planning and research, a process of doing more with less
"Green" buildings cost more	• no - sustainable building projects can be as cost effective as conventional ones
"Green" building is the architect's responsibility	• no - sustainable building design requires input from all stakeholders, including users, managers, designers and builders
"Green designs" look strange	• no - there is no such thing as a 'green' architecture look, and many sustainable buildings do not necessarily have a 'green' appearance
"Green" building information is not readily available	• no - a tremendous amount of information is now available (see list of resources at the end of this chapter)
"Green" buildings do not work	• no - green buildings provide better occupant satisfaction, are more efficient to operate and offer healthier work environments

Figure 8.2 Examples of common myths surrounding sustainable building design. (Data from [47].)

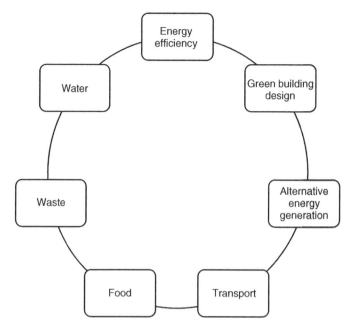

Figure 8.3 Elements of climate friendly healthcare buildings.

Principles for sustainable healthcare buildings

The *World Health Organization* and *Health Care Without Harm* have identified seven elements of a climate friendly hospital (Figure 8.3), which can, for the most part, also be applied to other healthcare buildings, such as general practices [15]. Interestingly, these components not only include elements that we would intuitively associate with a building, such as energy efficiency, alternative energy generation or green building design, but also factors that may initially appear to be 'outside' the remit of a building, such as transport, food and waste management (Chapters 6 and 9). This is a good example of systemic thinking in practice (Chapter 3).

Standards for new and old buildings

To help evaluate building designs, toolkits such as the *Guide for Sustainable Projects* by the American Institute of Architects or the *Achieving Excellence Design Evaluation Toolkit* (*AEDET Evolution*) use lists of statements in the key areas of impact, build quality and functionality [48, 49]. The *Centre for*

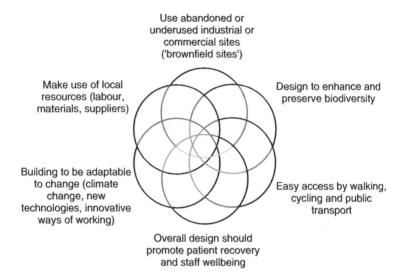

Figure 8.4   Aspects to consider when planning and designing new healthcare buildings. (Data from [52].)

Architecture and the Built Environment (CABE) advised the UK Government on architecture, urban design and public spaces from 1999 to 2011 (including sustainability and health) and has developed a wealth of material [50]. In its report *Future health: sustainable places for health and well-being*, CABE highlights the need for more integrated planning on the part of healthcare providers and professionals in terms of the types of services offered, how care is provided and the settings in which healthcare takes place [51]. Various aspects are worth considering when planning and designing new healthcare buildings and also when refitting or improving existing buildings to make them more sustainable [52]. Figure 8.4 gives an overview of issues that are particularly relevant for people involved planning and developing more sustainable buildings.

Various activities play a particular role in addressing these issues, particularly around optimising energy efficiency, using renewable sources of energy and looking at the way in which buildings and spaces are managed.

Optimising energy efficiency

With an increased focus on illness prevention and more care being provided in the community and in patients' homes, the greatest opportunities for carbon reduction and sustainability gains are currently around improving existing buildings. Many of the principles of increasing a building's performance apply to both new and existing ones. Making existing buildings more sustainable is a rapidly changing field and current initiatives, such as the *Design and Delivery of Robust Hospital Environments in a Changing Climate (De²RHECC)* project, explore practical and cost-effective strategies to help healthcare estates become more resilient to climate change whilst meeting current emissions targets [53]. Such projects help with devising strategies for effective refurbishment and reducing potential barriers for implementation.

Using energy more efficiently is an important easy first step [54]. Table 8.1 gives examples of financial and carbon savings that certain changes to the

Table 8.1 Examples of potential gains from carbon saving measures in buildings for NHS England. (Reproduced from [38] NHS Sustainable Development Unit. Saving Carbon, Improving Health: Carbon Reduction Strategy for England, with permission from the NHS Sustainable Development Unit.)

Carbon saving measures	CO_2 savings (tonnes CO_2/year)	Savings per year (£000 (US$ 000))
Decentralisation of hot water boilers in non-acute settings	10 612	2547 (3991)
Improve heating controls	26 551	3558 (5575)
Improve lighting controls	29 686	3770 (5907)
Energy efficient lighting	30 140	2743 (4298)
Voltage optimisation	29 364	2202 (3450)
Improve efficiency of chillers	7313	519 (813)
Roof insulation	25 928	1685 (2640)
Energy awareness campaign	92 549	5645 (8845)
Building management system optimisation	20 610	1154 (1808)
Improve insulation to pipe work, and in boiler house	11 195	616 (965)
A 1°C reduction in thermostat temperature	49 144	2605 (4081)
Improve efficiency of steam plant or hot water boiler plant	8933	465 (729)
Boiler replacement/optimisation for control centres	171	2 (3.1)
Wall insulation	25 928	207 (324)
Office electrical improvements	7957	32 (50)
Insulation	25 928	−156 (−244)
Biomass boiler	30 533	−1069 (−1675)

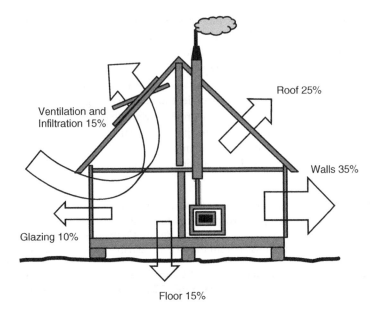

Ventilation and
Infiltration 15%

Roof 25%

Walls 35%

Glazing 10%

Floor 15%

Figure 8.5   Common heat losses from buildings.

running or design of a building can generate (Chapter 3 contains examples in other areas). Such data can be used to inform decisions about which measures make best financial sense and save most carbon. Particular gains can be achieved by improving a building's overall performance through, for example, reducing energy needs from lighting, heating and plug loads – and by optimising the way in which energy needs are monitored and controlled.

Improving building performance

One of the most effective ways of improving the performance of an existing building is to improve its shell, or *building envelope* (a term used for the structures of a building that separate the internal from the external environment), as heat loss through the shell can be considerable (Figure 8.5). Together with heating, ventilation and air conditioning (HVAC) systems, the building envelope plays a central role in maintaining the indoor environment and makes internal climate control possible.

An example of an effective and low-cost action involving the building envelope is to make sure that external doors are closed whenever possible, both during hot and cold periods. Improvements that need an initial investment include repairing leaking windows, doors and weather stripping.

Replacing windows with double- or, ideally, triple-glazed panes can cut heat loss through windows by half – but to make a sound business case, the 'return on investment' and building regulations need to be taken into account [19]. About one quarter of heat can escape through a non-insulated roof [55]. Insulating roofs, lofts, cavity walls and floors sufficiently is, therefore, crucial before trying to reduce the use of mechanical equipment, such as air conditioning. Using environmentally friendly construction materials is another important part of sustainable building.

Lighting

Asking staff to switch off unnecessary lighting carries little cost but is immediately effective. Real savings can also be achieved through a change in the type of lighting. Compact fluorescent and LED light bulbs use a quarter of the energy and last ten times longer than traditional incandescent filament bulbs [56]. Occupancy sensors can help to improve energy use in areas that are frequently unoccupied. Automatic dimming or bi-/multilevel switching (in which alternate rows, fixtures or lamps are separately circuited and independently controlled) can reduce energy bills by up to around 60% [57]. Daylight sensors in public areas and patient rooms with plenty of natural light can ensure that lights are being switched off when not needed. A 'downtime lighting' policy can help reduce overall lighting levels.

Heating, ventilation and air conditioning (HVAC)

Central heating, ventilation and air conditioning systems contribute to a high proportion of a building's energy use – and energy bill. Low cost and high return activities include checking, calibrating and adjusting thermostats that heat or cool different parts of a building. Settings can be adjusted to account for different levels of occupancy. One energy saving measure is to adjust our expectations of room temperature. Research into 'thermal comfort' shows that a remarkably wide range of factors contribute to whether or not we feel comfortable with the temperature of an internal environment [58]. Many medical interiors are maintained above 23°C. Keeping offices at 19 or 20°C will mean that some staff need to wear slightly warmer clothing, but patients, who arrive dressed for the outdoors, are unlikely to complain. Conversely, there is usually little need for air conditioning to bring temperatures below 25°C.

To work to their best effect and continue to generate savings, HVAC units need regular maintenance, which includes cleaning and replacing filters, inspecting pipes and pipe insulation for any damage, and conducting replacements or repairs as necessary. Making sure that chillers and heat transfer coils, air conditioners and heat pumps are cleaned and serviced regularly ensures optimum performance. Although such measures are usually obvious to people working in estates departments, they are also relevant for other healthcare workers, in that early reporting of faulty HVAC units and reducing operator-generated energy wastage potentially makes a big difference in improving building efficiency.

Plug loads

Office equipment, medical apparatus and other appliances (such as lifts, scanners or surgical equipment) consume considerable amounts of energy. There are many ways to reduce energy consumption from these *plug loads*. Stand-by consumption, also called *phantom* or *vampire loads*, can leak unexpectedly large amounts of energy. Unplugging non-essential equipment and providing accessible power strips is low cost and easy to implement. *Standby-savers* are power strips that automatically turn off peripherals such as scanners, monitors and printers when users switch off the main computer. Purchasing devices that consume less energy than standard models (certified, for example, by *ENERGY STAR®* in the United States or the *Energy Saving Trust®* in the United Kingdom) is usually less immediate and will incur some costs, but has the potential to reduce an organisation's energy bill. Some appliances, including medical equipment such as MRI scanners and automated patient monitoring systems, often have power management settings. Using these settings during working hours and switching off these devices when they are not in use can generate substantial savings over time. Replacing standard cathode ray tube (CRT) computer monitors with LED monitors will reduce consumption by 25–60%.

Using metering

Power control tools are now available in many locations and can be linked to so-called 'smart metering', which is a way to monitor energy use through an integrated way of power management. Electricity monitors record the flow of electricity into buildings and transmit that information wirelessly to a digital display placed in a prominent position (like the manager's desk). By switching off as many appliances as possible, users can determine the background energy needs of a building for things like fridges and servers. It is then possible to see immediately when appliances are being left on unnecessarily at the end of the day. Just *having* the monitor will save money. For example, in a Dutch housing scheme, houses were randomised to be fitted with energy monitoring displays in either the basement or the porch – and those with the display in the porch used 15% less energy. The latest energy monitor models include the facility to download usage patterns to computer via a USB port.

Continuous commissioning

Verifying that in a new building all the subsystems such as heating, plumbing, lighting, controls and building envelops achieve the necessary requirement is called *building commissioning*. This process helps ensure that buildings meet the occupiers' needs at the optimum of cost and performance. Traditionally, this course of action takes place before a building is handed over, but to get the best from buildings, this commissioning should be an integral part of the building process, from design and construction to operation – a process known as *continuous commissioning* [59]. If applied appropriately, continuous commissioning can deliver substantial benefits in terms of energy consumption, operating costs and reduced environmental impact while providing buildings that are of better quality, more comfortable and run at lower costs. Many architects and estate managers now rate continuous commissioning among the key processes when it comes to making buildings more sustainable.

Continuous commissioning may take the form of a continuing project that includes activities such as developing improved control schedules, making changes to automatic programmes, estimating potential performance changes and energy savings, and conducting regular performance analyses [59]. In other words, continuous commissioning is about making sure that everything works properly – and that it does so all day and every day.

Using renewable and alternative sources of energy

Renewable sources of energy, such as wind, hydroelectric, biomass, geothermal and solar power, are increasingly available for use in the health sector. The buying power of health services can encourage investment in such alternatives. Good financial reasons, and concern for reputation, often exist for committing to international and national incentives that aim to implement lower carbon operations, such as the *Carbon Reduction Commitment – Energy Efficiency Scheme (CRC-EES)* in the United Kingdom [60]. Healthcare organisations may even have the opportunity to generate renewable energy in or around their facilities. This may not only reduce carbon emissions but also create additional income that can be invested in other sustainability improvements or patient care (Case study 8.6).

The *UK Partnership for Renewables* has additional information and examples of how making better use of renewable energy can work in

Case study 8.6   Kentish Town Integrated Health Centre, London, UK [61]

The Camden Primary Care Trust (UK) built its new Kentish Town Integrated Health Centre with an energy reduction design, engineered to be more than 12 times more efficient than its previous health centre. The design of the building aimed to assist health promotion and address inequalities while minimising the need for acute services. Integral design features included natural light, passive cooling and solar panels. The purpose of the building is flexible, with rooms being able to adapt to possible changes in future demand and equipped to be used by various healthcare staff. 'Hot desking' is efficient in terms of space allocation and usability, and communal spaces for staff promote a multidisciplinary approach to delivering primary care. Communal meeting rooms can also be subdivided into six spaces, which allows hosting antenatal classes, yoga groups and private functions, which helps increase the community's cohesion. The waiting area has a café that is run by a local business and provides Internet access points. The self-service check-in features 'health pods' where people can measure their blood pressure, weight and height to save time before they see a health professional and improve data collection. The centre also has 'green' travel and waste management plans and is easily accessible through public transport. There is no parking except for disabled access bays, and private use of cars is discouraged.

practice [62]. Using or creating renewable energy, or both, often needs health services to invest money up front. This investment may become cost neutral over time, as the potential for savings later on can be substantial, particularly if services or equipment are purchased in bulk to get better deals. Solar thermal energy generation for heating water, for example, can provide great opportunities in the health sector, because many healthcare providers such as hospitals need hot water almost all the time (Case study 8.7).

Access to reliable energy is important for running healthcare facilities effectively but can pose a challenge – in particular in rural areas of lower income countries. Diesel generators often provide the necessary energy, but these are expensive and polluting, and they often cause high carbon emissions. Such generators are always at risk of breaking down, and unless backup generators or alternative forms of energy generation are available, procedures may need to be cancelled and services are disrupted when energy supplies are down. For this reason, low-maintenance alternative energy can

Case study 8.7   Using solar panels in a UK hospital [61]

The roof of the Princess Alexandra Hospital in Harlow, UK, which serves a quarter of a million patients over five sites, has a large array of solar hot water panels on its roof. The project arose from a need to reduce energy costs, which were set to rise from £1 million (US$ 1.6 million) to £1.5 million (US$ 2.4 million). In 2007, the hospital secured a grant of £400 000 (US$ 641 500) from the Department of Health's Energy Fund to install two new energy efficient boilers and low-maintenance solar panels. Solar water heating systems that use free heat from the sun warm up the site's water prior to it reaching the boilers, so that the boilers have to do significantly less work. This has resulted in a 50% reduction in the number of times the boilers have to fire up to heat the water and, at optimum operation levels, 40–50% of the building's hot water requirements are met by the solar panel's output. The savings achieved by the solar panels and new efficient boilers equated to a reduction of 8000 m^3 of gas and 16 tonnes carbon dioxide per year. Bill Dickson, Energy Manager at the hospital, was quoted as saying: 'This is a project that could be replicated on any south-facing NHS building that has a high demand for hot water. The payback time for the project is between ten and twelve years; however, this may become considerably less if energy prices continue to rise. We are keen that other trusts, which may be scratching their heads about how to cut their energy costs at a time when we are all under financial pressure, see what we have achieved and consider how they might follow suit'.

be very attractive for healthcare provision in areas with limited electricity or fuel, as Case study 8.8 demonstrates.

Sustainability management of buildings in context

A useful starting point for making energy savings and reducing carbon emissions is to measure direct and indirect energy usage routinely. Ideally, such data are collected centrally. In the United Kingdom, for example, the *NHS Information Centre* routinely collects data through its *Estate Returns Information Collection (ERIC)*, which informs benchmarking and setting targets for efficiency improvements in terms of energy use, travel and procurement. In many healthcare settings, public reporting of energy use and efficiency has already become the norm. All NHS sites above a certain size are legally bound to put on view a *Display Energy Certificate* that summarises

---

Case study 8.8   Solar energy in Rwanda

Rural health clinics in Rwanda opted for solar energy, with support from *Partners in Health* and in collaboration with the *Solar Electric Light Fund (SELF)* [63]. In these clinics, solar–diesel hybrid systems now provide 90% of the power, backed up by diesel generators during rain or particularly heavy use. Solar energy is now the main source of energy used for vaccine refrigeration, remote satellite communication and computerised patient record keeping. LED lighting, sterilisation devices, blood analysis machines, centrifuges or portable X-ray machines can also all be powered through solar power.

---

building efficiency, which is useful for allowing comparison between different sites. Such public reporting should become more and more common, so that healthcare organisations can come under scrutiny and be accountable for the way they manage their buildings and energy use.

Sharing best practice

Sustainable building is an area where a tremendous amount of experience exists already. Yet it is also a field from where innovative designs and initiatives constantly emerge. Organisations and initiatives, such as *Healthcare Without Harm* (www.noharm.org), the *Learning Network for Sustainable Healthcare Building (SHINE)* (www.shine-network.org.uk) or the *Commission for Architecture and the Built Environment (CABE)*, promote good practice in carbon reduction. Their information and guidance can be invaluable for anyone involved in trying to make healthcare buildings and spaces greener [50]. The *Green Guide for Health Care* established in 2002 as part of a project of the non-profit organisations *Health Care Without Harm (HCWH)* and the *Center for Maximum Potential Building Systems (CMPBS)* is a useful starting point, as it informs on designing and building healthcare environments that are environmentally friendly, increase sustainability and reduce or even produce zero carbon emissions [64]. Further sources of information are listed at the end of this chapter.

Investing to save

When thinking about investing in energy or building projects it is important to consider *whole life costing* (sometimes also called 'cradle to grave' or 'womb to tomb' costing). This type of costing needs to not only consider financial price tags but also the broader as well as longer-term social and environmental costs [65]. Although environmental and social costs are often difficult to quantify, estimations can still be valuable. When calculating the whole life cost, considering replacement, disposal, depreciation, renewal and rehabilitation costs in addition to costs relating to design and planning, constructing, operating and maintenance is crucial. Further information about whole life costing in evaluating the carbon impacts of building design is widely available, for example from the *Carbon Trust* in its document *Low carbon refurbishment of buildings – Management guide* and other resources listed later in this chapter [66].

Local solutions and working in partnership

Although various low carbon building and energy solutions are available, their suitability for particular health settings depends on the local situation. Heat generation is a good example where the needs of larger urban hospitals vary from those of smaller rural buildings. When planning to implement new forms of heat generation it is worth investigating possible collaboration with the local community, making use of partnership solutions such as *District Energy Schemes* or *Community Heating Schemes*. District heating is a way of distributing heat produced in a central location for commercial and residential users in the wider community, usually for heating spaces, water or both. Evidence suggests that combining district heating with *Combined Heat and Power* (also called CHPDH) can be an effective and practical method with a comparatively low carbon footprint [67]. While an ordinary thermal power station can have an energy efficiency of around 20–35%, facilities that are able to recover unused heat can be up to 80% energy efficient [68].

The future for sustainable buildings

Although initiatives for 'greener' buildings and energy use are not new, sustainable construction and design is a rapidly changing field. Creating buildings in the past has focused around function, comfort and budget, and much less on how well they fit with the natural environment [69]. Traditionally, buildings have also been created 'for the moment', with little consideration for the needs of future generations. A number of building concepts have emerged that challenge traditional ways of building design. By using innovative strategies and technologies, such buildings seek to integrate and restore the natural environment, thereby becoming more autonomous when it comes to using resources such as water or electricity [69].

For example, architects with an interest in sustainable building will often try to include *regenerative design* features in their projects, such as solar panelling that provides enough energy to power the building – or even a surplus that provides energy for the wider community. This is a relatively new field (particularly in the area of healthcare), but where such features are successfully implemented, buildings have the capacity to *generate* net resources instead *consuming* them. The healthcare sector has an opportunity to move in this direction and to set an important example by creating buildings that not only 'do no harm' but that become true 'healing' places – both from a patient care and an environmental point of view. Such buildings and spaces have great potential to create positive effects for local communities and the wider population – and thereby contribute to a fairer and stronger society [15, 69].

Building a more sustainable future

Buildings and spaces play an important role within the provision of healthcare – and will continue to do so for the foreseeable future. Plenty of opportunities exist to make existing buildings more efficient, not only saving carbon and money but often at the same time also improving the quality of life for patients and staff. Identifying the 'low hanging fruit' – those actions that cost little but have a big impact in terms of financial and carbon savings – is often the best first step to creating better buildings.

In this chapter we have reviewed how buildings and available green spaces affect health. It follows that, in addition to environmental and financial benefits, making healthcare buildings more sustainable can improve patient care and the quality of life for healthcare staff. As we have demonstrated, there are many ways to increase sustainability: we can make changes to the buildings themselves and we can also change the way in which we use them. The biggest sustainability gains, though, are to be made somewhere else: in the area of resource use and procurement. And this is what the next chapter is all about.

Useful sources for further information

A selection of websites that contain a wealth of additional information and are useful resources for keeping up with latest developments in the field of buildings and energy is given in Box 8.1.

Box 8.1 Sources of additional information and resources

- American Institute of Architects, Committee on the Environment, http://network.aia.org/committeeontheenvironment/home/
- Carbon Trust, www.carbontrust.co.uk
- Centre for Sustainable Healthcare, www.sustainablehealthcare.org.uk
- ENERGY STAR®, www.energystar.gov
- Energy Saving Trust, www.energysavingtrust.org.uk
- Green Guide for Healthcare, www.gghc.org
- Healthcare Without Harm, www.noharm.org
- International Living Future Institute™, https://ilbi.org/lbc
- Learning Network for Sustainable Healthcare Building (SHINE), www.shine-network.org.uk
- NHS Sustainable Development Unit (SDU), www.sdu.nhs.uk
- UK Department of Energy and Climate Change, www.decc.gov.uk
- US Green Building Council, http://www.usgbc.org
- US Department of Energy, www.energy.gov

Key actions

Person

- Turn thermostats down a few degrees in winter and up in summer – even a slight shift can create significant energy savings.
- Use resources (such as water and energy) sparingly and re-use and recycle where possible.

Practice

- Make reviewing energy and carbon management a board-level activity in your healthcare organisation.
- Encourage a broader approach to sustainability (including transport, delivery of service and community engagement) when making decisions about design and build of healthcare facilities.

- Conduct regular board-level reviews of performance in energy efficiency and carbon reduction, and report these in regular intervals to staff, the public and other stakeholders.
- Create an infrastructure for action, such as a committee to spearhead organisation-wide sustainability measures (to include baseline emissions, developing priorities and preparing guidelines for environmental initiatives).
- Adopt facility-wide energy efficiency and conservation practices and incentives (for example, fitting occupancy sensitive lighting, using energy monitors etc.).
- Install energy efficient lighting and occupancy sensor switches throughout your facilities.
- Establish the current carbon footprint of the building and set carbon reduction targets for any refurbishments.
- When retrofitting old buildings or developing a new build, consult building occupants and key stakeholders at the beginning of the process and ensure project buy-in from the design team and site workers.
- Appoint a carbon champion at an early stage of a project to maintain a focus on energy use implications of design decisions.
- Use a whole life cost analysis to evaluate low carbon systems and components.
- Ensure high quality commissioning for energy efficiency, allocating a specific budget for the purpose.

Policy

- Use your professional influence to advocate for sustainability causes and team up with colleagues to press policy makers.
- Support broader aspects of sustainability in the built environment, including the use of local and regional materials (reducing transport energy), using salvaged and recycled materials (reducing energy otherwise expended on new production) and supporting toxic-free products and manufacturing processes.
- Replace energy measurements with carbon measurements as the main target for reductions.

References

1. Heathcote, E. and Jencks, C. (eds) (2010) *The Architecture of Hope: Maggie's Cancer Caring Centres*. Frances Lincoln, London.

2. Ulrich, R.S. (1991) Effects of interior design on wellness: theory and recent scientific research. *Journal of health care interior design*, **3**, 97–109.
3. Kirklin, D. and Richardson, R. (2003) *The healing environment: without and within*. Royal College of Physicians, London.
4. Thompson, J.D. and Goldin, G. (1995) *The hospital: A social and architectural history*. Yale University Press, New Haven, CT.
5. The Center for Health Design – Evidence-based Design Accreditation and Certification (EDAC) [Internet]. http://www.healthdesign.org/edac/about [accessed 27 February 2012].
6. Wagenaar, C. (2006) *The architecture of hospitals*. NAi Publishers, Rotterdam, The Netherlands.
7. Enhancing the Healing Environment Programme (Home) [Internet].http://www.enhancingthehealingenvironment.org.uk/default.asp [accessed 14 February 2012].
8. Ranking Web of World Hospitals (Home) [Internet]. Available from: http://hospitals.webometrics.info/about_rank.html [accessed 28 Oct 2011].
9. Johnson, S.J. (2010) *Assertive Community Treatment: Evidence-based Practice or Managed Recovery*. Transaction Publishers.
10. Elkan, R., Kendrick, D., Dewey, M. *et al.* (2001) Effectiveness of home based support for older people: systematic review and meta-analysis Commentary: When, where, and why do preventive home visits. *British Medical Journal*, **323** (7315), 719.
11. Bodenheimer, T., Wagner, E.H. and Grumbach, K. (2002) Improving primary care for patients with chronic illness: the chronic care model, Part 2. *Journal of the American Medical Association*, **288** (15), 1909–1914.
12. Bueno, H., Ross, J.S., Wang, Y. *et al.* (2010) Trends in length of stay and short-term outcomes among Medicare patients hospitalized for heart failure, 1993–2006. *Journal of the American Medical Association*, **303** (21), 2141–2147.
13. Cargill, Y., Martel, M-J., Society of Obstetricians and Gynaecologists of Canada (2007) Postpartum maternal and newborn discharge. *Journal of Obstetrics and Gynaecology Canada*, **29** (4), 357–363.
14. Wilson, E. (1990) *Biophilia*. Harvard University Press, Cambridge, MA.
15. World Health Organization and Healthcare Without Harm (2009) Healthy hospitals, healthy planet, healthy people: Addressing climate change in healthcare settings [Internet]. http://www.who.int/globalchange/publications/healthcare_settings/en/index.html [accessed 2 August 2011].
16. Guenther, R. and Vittori, G. (2008) *Sustainable healthcare architecture*. John Wiley and Sons Ltd, Chichester.
17. Stern, A., MacRae, S., Gerteis, M. *et al.* (2003) Understanding the consumer perspective to improve design quality. *Journal of Architectural and Planning Research*, **20** (1), 16–28.
18. Maller, C., Townsend, M., Pryor, A., Brown, P. and St, Leger L. (2006) Healthy nature healthy people: "contact with nature" as an upstream health promotion intervention for populations. *Health Promotion International*, **21** (1), 45–54.
19. Ulrich, R. (1984) View through a window may influence recovery from surgery. *Science*, 1984 **224**, 420–421.

20. The Construction Information Service (2005) Improving the patient experience. A place to die with dignity: creating a supportive environment [Internet].http://products.ihs.com/cis/Doc.aspx?AuthCode=&DocNum=280078 [accessed 14 February 2012].
21. Guy's and St Thomas' NHS Foundation Trust – Savannah Ward [Internet]. http://www.guysandstthomas.nhs.uk/our-services/wards/savannah.aspx [accessed 14 February 2012].
22. Stevenson, F. and Humphris, M. (2007) A post occupancy evaluation of the Dundee Maggie Centre [Internet]. 2007. Available from: http://sust.org/pdf/new_maggiecentre.pdf (accessed 4 February 2012)
23. Maggie's Cancer Caring Centres (Home) [Internet]. http://www.maggiescentres.org/ [accessed 4 February 2012].
24. Glasgow Homoeopathic Hospital (Home) [Internet]. http://ghh.info/welcome.htm [accessed 4 February 2012].
25. Institute of Rural Health – Research reports [Internet]. http://www.ruralhealth.ac.uk/publications/research-publications.php [accessed 11 September 2011].
26. UK Faculty of Public Health (2010) New FPH mental health report calls for more use of walks in parks to treat mental illness [Internet]. http://www.fph.org.uk/new_fph_mental_health_report_calls_for_more_use_of_walks_in_parks_to_treat_mental_illness [accessed 29 October 2011].
27. Bird, W. (2007) Natural thinking [Internet]. http://www.rspb.org.uk/Images/naturalthinking_tcm9-161856.pdf [accessed 29 October 2011].
28. Yerrell, P. (2008) National evaluation of BTCV's Green Gym. School of Health and Social Care, Oxford Brookes University, Oxford.
29. The Blue Gym (Home) [Internet]. http://www.bluegym.org.uk/ [accessed 4 February 2012].
30. Depledge, M.H. and Bird, W.J. (2009) The Blue Gym: health and wellbeing from our coasts. *Marine Pollution Bulletin*, **58** (7), 947–948.
31. Sustainable Development Commission (2008) Health, Place and Nature [Internet]. http://www.sd-commission.org.uk/publications.php?id=712 [accessed 4 September 2011].
32. Lachowycz, K. and Jones, A.P. (2011) Greenspace and obesity: a systematic review of the evidence. *Obesity Review*, **12** (5), e183–189.
33. RSPB – Health: - nature improves your fitness and reduces stress [Internet]. http://www.rspb.org.uk/ourwork/policy/health/index.aspx [accessed 25 November 2011].
34. Maas, J., Verheij, R.A., de Vries, S., Spreeuwenberg, P., Schellevis, F.G. and Groenewegen, P.P. (2009) Morbidity is related to a green living environment. *Journal of Epidemiology & Community Health*, **63**, 967–973.
35. Kaplan, R. and Kaplan S. (1989) *The Experience of Nature: A Psychological Perspective*. Cambridge University Press.
36. The Retreat York – Therapy in the open air [Internet]. http://www.theretreatyork.org.uk/news/archive-news/therapy-in-the-open-air.html [accessed 19 August 2011].

37. NHS Sustainable Development Unit – Are you a Good Corporate Citizen? Buildings: Key areas [Internet]. http://www.corporatecitizen.nhs.uk/pages/buildings.html [accessed 5 November 2011].

38. NHS Sustainable Development Unit, (2009) Saving Carbon, Improving Health: Carbon Reduction Strategy for England. NHS Sustainable Development Unit, Cambridge. 2009.

39. Berners-Lee, M. (2010) *How Bad Are Bananas?: The carbon footprint of everything*. Profile Books, London.

40. ODAC: The Oil Depletion Analysis Centre (Home) [Internet]. http://www.odacinfo.org/ [accessed 19 August 2011].

41. NHS Sustainable Development Unit – Energy and Carbon Management [Internet]. http://www.sdu.nhs.uk/documents/publications/1234888949_zfGK_energy_and_carbon_management.pdf [accessed 19 August 2011].

42. US Green Building Council (USGBC) – What LEED Is [Internet]. http://www.usgbc.org/DisplayPage.aspx?CMSPageID=1988 [accessed 5 November 2011].

43. BREEAM – What is BREEAM? [Internet]. http://www.breeam.org/page.jsp?id=66 [accessed 20 August 2011].

44. Green Building Council Australia (GBCA) – Green Star: Healthcare v1 (Rating tools) [Internet]. http://www.gbca.org.au/green-star/green-star-healthcare-v1/1936.htm [accessed 5 November 2011].

45. Abu Dhabi Urban Planning Council (UPC) – Estidama [Internet]. http://estidama.org/estidama-and-pearl-rating-system.aspx?lang=en-US [accessed 5 November 2011].

46. Practice Greenhealth – Energy Impact Calculator [Internet]. http://practicegreenhealth.org/tools-resources/energy-impact-calculator [accessed 28 February 2012].

47. Roberts, G. Top 10 Green-Building Myths. *Healthcare Design Magazine*, 2003 **3**, 26–30.

48. The American Institute of Architects – AIA Guide for Sustainable Projects [Internet]. Available from: http://info.aia.org/aia/sustainabilityguide.cfm [accessed 4 September 2011].

49. Department of Health – Achieving Excellence Design Evaluation Toolkit (AEDET Evolution): http://www.dh.gov.uk/en/Publicationsandstatistics/Publications/PublicationsPolicyAndGuidance/DH_082089 [accessed 4 September 2011].

50. CABE (The Commission for Architecture and the Built Environment) [Internet]. http://webarchive.nationalarchives.gov.uk/20110118095356/http://www.cabe.org.uk/home [accessed 21 November 2011].

51. CABE (2009) Future health: Sustainable places for health and well-being [Internet]. http://webarchive.nationalarchives.gov.uk/20110118095356/http://www.cabe.org.uk/files/future-health-full-report_0.pdf [accessed 21 November 2011].

52. Sustainable Development Commission (2005) Healthy Futures #3: Buildings and Sustainable Development [Internet]. http://www.sd-commission.org.uk/publications.php?id=246 [accessed 4 September 2011].

53. Engineering and Physical Sciences Research Council – Design and delivery of robust hospital environments in a changing climate [Internet]. http://www-edc. eng.cam.ac.uk/robusthospitals/Project/ [accessed 25 November 2011].
54. World Health Organization – Health in the Green Economy: co-benefits to health of climate change mitigation. http://www.who.int/hia/hgebrief_health.pdf [accessed 31 July 2012].
55. Energy Saving Trust – Roof and loft insulation [Internet]. http://www. energysavingtrust.org.uk/In-your-home/Roofs-floors-walls-and-windows/Roof-and-loft-insulation [accessed 14 February 2012].
56. Energy Saving Trust – Energy Saving Light Bulbs [Internet]. http://www. energysavingtrust.org.uk/Home-improvements-and-products/Lighting [accessed 10 September 2011].
57. Lighting Controls Association (2007) Bi-level Switching Study Demonstrates Energy Savings [Internet]. http://lightingcontrolsassociation.org/bi-level-switching-study-demonstrates-energy-savings/ [accessed 10 September 2011].
58. Nicol, F., Humphreys, M. and Roaf S. (2012) *Adaptive Thermal Comfort*: *Principles and Practice.* Routledge.
59. US Department of Energy (2002) Continuous Commissioning Guidebook for Federal Energy Managers [Internet]. http://www1.eere.energy.gov/femp/ program/om_guidebook.html [accessed 5 November 2011].
60. UK CRC (Carbon Reduction Committee) – CRCEES [Internet]. http:// www.ukcrc.co.uk/articles/crcees.htm [accessed 5 November 2011].
61. NHS Sustainable Development Unit – Case studies [Internet]. http:// www.sdu.nhs.uk/publications-resources/case-studies.aspx [accessed 28 October 2011].
62. Partnerships for Renewables (Home) [Internet]. http://www.pfr.co.uk/pfr/2/ About-Us/ [accessed 4 August 2011].
63. Solar Electric Light Fund – Projects: Rwanda [Internet]. [cited 2011 Sep 6]. Available from: http://www.self.org/rwanda.shtml [accessed 6 September 2011].
64. GGHC – About GGHC: Objectives [Internet]. http://www.gghc.org/about .objectives.php [accessed 21 August 2011].
65. Charlesworth, A., Gray, A., Pencheon, D. and Stern, N. (2011) Assessing the health benefits of tackling climate change. *British Medical Journal*, **343**, d6520.
66. Carbon Trust – Low carbon refurbishment of buildings: management guide [Internet]. http://www.carbontrust.co.uk/Publications/pages/publicationdetail .aspx?id=CTV038 [accessed 3 September 2011].
67. Claverton Group – Carbon footprints of various sources of heat : CHPDH comes out lowest [Internet].http://www.claverton-energy.com/carbon-footprints-of-various-sources-of-heat-chpdh-comes-out-lowest.html [accessed 3 September 2011].
68. US Department of Energy – Fossil Energy: How Turbine Power Plants Work [Internet]. http://fossil.energy.gov/programs/powersystems/turbines/turbines _howitworks.html [accessed 3 September 2011].
69. Whole Building Design Guide (2010) Living, Regenerative, and Adaptive Buildings [Internet]. http://www.wbdg.org/resources/livingbuildings.php [accessed 5 November 2011].

Chapter 9 **Resource stewardship**

In this chapter

- Putting sustainable procurement into perspective
- Using water more efficiently
- Managing waste

In this chapter, we take a look at the story of resources in the health sector, from sourcing them, to using them and finally disposing of them. Our focus is on three areas that have a particular impact on sustainability: procuring goods and services, managing water and reducing waste. In England, the National Health Service (NHS) spends around £20 billion (US$ 32 billion) every year on goods, medicines, medical supplies, food, computers, stationery and services, resulting in a carbon footprint estimated at over 11 million tonnes a year [1, 2]. Once they have been used, many material things, such as dressings, syringes or broken equipment, will often end up as waste. But there is really no such thing as *waste*, so what we are really talking about is *wasted resources*, such as nutrients, recyclable materials and energy. By disposing of waste we will not make it go away – we only shift it to another place. Also, managing waste does not come cheaply. In the UK NHS the costs for disposing of waste amounted to a profligate £83 million (US$ 133 million) in 2009/2010 [3]. Some types of health sector waste are more expensive to manage than others. For example, in the United Kingdom it costs around £370 (US$ 593) to dispose of one tonne of clinical waste. This is defined as waste that consists wholly or partly of human tissue, blood, bodily fluids, drugs, swabs, used syringes and similar items, all of which may cause infection to any person coming into contact with it; it is typically disposed of through incineration, which itself results in pollution. In comparison, disposing of non-clinical waste comes much cheaper at £70 (US$ 112) per tonne [4]. It is *crucial*, therefore, to make sure that such waste is correctly segregated, reducing both environmental impact and costs [5].

Sustainable Healthcare, First Edition. Knut Schroeder, Trevor Thompson, Kathleen Frith and David Pencheon.
© 2013 John Wiley & Sons, Ltd. Published 2013 by John Wiley & Sons, Ltd.

Health systems are also major consumers of another ubiquitous resource: water. Without water, there is no healthcare. Where water supplies are scarce, health services appreciate the value of water. But in the temperate zones, where water is still relatively plentiful, its cost is rarely taken into account and we often take supplies for granted. However, sourcing water and managing the resulting sewage has substantial cost implications. For instance, in 2007/2008, the NHS in England spent £145 million (US$ 232 million) on buying and disposing of water [6]. Pumping water requires energy, and treating drain water is four times more carbon intensive than supplying the water in the first instance – unless we consider bottled water, which has up to 2000 times the carbon impact of tap water [2].

These figures and examples illustrate the magnitude of resource use in the health sector – and the opportunities that we can create for reducing waste and costs by managing resources better. So in this chapter, we outline some of the harmful effects of current practice in these areas and demonstrate the positive effects that can arise from adopting more sustainable ways of doing things.

Procurement in perspective

Procurement contributes a hefty 60% of the total NHS carbon footprint in England [7]. Pharmaceuticals and medical equipment generate around half of these procurement emissions (Figure 9.1), which is comparable to the combined carbon impacts from health-related travel and building energy. To better understand procurement and its effects on resources, we need to appreciate the journey that materials and products take during their 'lifetime'.

Resource cycles in healthcare

The complete consumption process – including sourcing, producing, consuming, recycling and disposing of materials and products – forms the so-called *resource cycle* (Figure 9.2; see also Chapter 3).

The health sector plays an important part in the global resource cycle, as the following general examples illustrate. For health services to work effectively, they depend on certain resources, such as raw materials for medicines, fossil fuels for heating buildings or transporting patients, energy for running hospitals, water and various chemicals. Making use of these resources leads to substantial greenhouse gas emissions and various forms of waste – on a large scale. And this creates opportunities for action. For example, healthcare organisations can make their resource cycles more effective by reducing

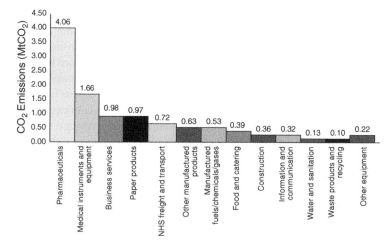

Figure 9.1 Breakdown of NHS England 2004 procurement emissions. (Reproduced from [7] http://www.sdu.nhs.uk/documents/publications/1263313924_jgyW_nhs_england_carbon_emissions_carbon_footprinting_r .pdf, with permission from the NHS Sustainable Development Unit.)

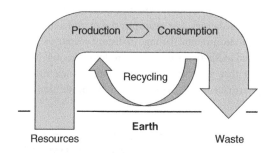

Figure 9.2 The resource cycle.

the *net use* of resources or increasing their 'lifetime' by recycling materials and products (which of course also comes at a cost, as it still requires a certain amount of energy and resources, but this cost is usually considerably smaller). Where resources used by the health sector finally end up in landfill sites, they leave the cycle and are usually impossible (or at least impractical) to recover. In most cases, they will be 'lost forever'. So what practical actions can we take?

An important first step is to think about the process of buying. As we know, health systems routinely purchase medicines, food, chemicals, electrical equipment, office supplies and energy. Such processes require a succession of important decisions, from *what* and *where* to buy to *how much* to buy. It follows that making decisions about procuring such items sustainably can be difficult. What if a product can be fully recycled but lasts for only a year? Would this mean that this is better in sustainability and financial terms than obtaining one that cannot be recycled but lasts for many years? And would it be better to buy an energy-efficient piece of equipment which has been produced in a far-off location than a product that needs more energy to run, but has been produced more locally? At present, such decisions are often hampered by the difficulty of not always knowing the true carbon footprint of common procured items, such as pharmaceuticals. Yet there has been progress in this area, which is covered later in this chapter [8]. To make genuinely more sustainable decisions, we need the relevant knowledge and tools on a case by case basis. And to achieve this we require local standards that are informed by recognised national and international guidelines and backed by a systematic research programme. In the following sections we look at a few selected areas to show how this can work in practice. Procuring more locally is often a good start. Case study 9.1 gives an example of how more local procurement can be encouraged.

But just buying more locally is not enough. We also need to be aware of the wider supply and disposal chain, especially when it comes to food (Chapter 6) and medicines. For example, the manufacture of products may be the cause of environmental damage in distant countries. And many people who flush unused medicines through the toilet seem oblivious to (or plainly ignore) the fact that wastewater treatment plants are often ineffective in eliminating pharmaceuticals, which can have subtle damaging effects on

---

Case study 9.1   Supporting local businesses [9]

The *Groundwork Environmental Business Services (EBS)* in the United Kingdom supports local economic development by helping local businesses tender for contracts with the NHS. Environmental advisers help organisations not only with conducting resource efficiency reviews and developing environmental policies but also with implementing environmental management systems and sustainable procurement. This programme has been shown to be of considerable value not only for organisations but also to suppliers; for example, a small fruit and vegetable distributor was part of this programme and as a result won a prestigious health and safety award as well as a number of lucrative contracts.

aquatic systems, such as the feminisation of fish populations or harming vital microbes and invertebrates in the soil [10]. This is the growing area of *ecopharmacovigilance*, which is concerned with the science and activities associated with detecting, evaluating, understanding and preventing adverse effects of pharmaceuticals in the natural environment [11]. So it is easy to see how *any* clinical or procurement decisions in the health sector – such as writing a script for an antibiotic or buying medical equipment – can have more far-reaching implications than we perhaps may imagine.

Safer purchase and use of chemicals

Chemical elements and compounds have been linked to serious illnesses such as cancer, asthma, infertility and developmental delay [12]. Some of these substances pollute the indoor environment and others, like dioxin or mercury, are leading to global environmental health concerns. A systematic review estimated that 375 000 people died globally from occupational particulates in 2004 [13]. Chemicals are also present in many healthcare environments and include disinfectants, sterilisers, chemotherapy substances, pesticides for controlling pests on site, chemicals in thermometers and medical devices, cleaning agents and agents used for controlling disease vectors, such as malaria [14]. Consequently, health services can play an important role in improving the safety of patients, staff, communities and the environment by becoming more aware of the ingredients of chemical products and cleaning agents and by switching to safer alternatives (for example those that are easily biodegradable) whenever possible [15].

Better medicine procurement and management

An independent study commissioned by the UK Department of Health found that unused prescriptions cost the NHS at least £300 million (US$ 481 million) a year, of which £150 million (US$ 240 million) was avoidable [16]. This 2010 report concluded that using medicines effectively could generate up to £500 million (US$ 801 million) of extra value in the five therapeutic areas of asthma, diabetes, high blood pressure, vascular disease and schizophrenia. To make better use of medicines and avoid waste, the Kings Fund suggests the following actions [17]:

- Engaging people in the decisions about their medicines.
- Providing targeted support for patients starting new therapies.
- Better use of medicines use reviews (MURs) and prescription interventions.
- Better communication between health professionals.
- Better systems for managing repeat prescribing.

- Better systems for managing medicines in care homes.
- Better management of medicines at the end-of-life care period.
- Further research into optimising waste management.

To prevent medication from becoming out of date before it is issued, new stocking systems for pharmacies have been developed. For instance, 'stockless' pharmacies optimise their stock management and reduce costs by using quick notices to indicate that stock depletion requires new stock to be ordered, which is then followed by a fast procurement response. One of the most important aspects of more effective medicines management is better prescribing, which features in more detail in Chapter 5.

Medical devices and ICT

Medical devices are big business, turning over an estimated US$ 312 billion (£195 billion) worldwide in 2011 [18]. Unfortunately, they are not always produced under ethical conditions. For example, around 10 million surgical instruments enter the United Kingdom every year from northern Pakistan, where most of the 50 000 manual labourers work 12 hours a day for well below the living wage – many of them children [19]. In addition to medical devices, modern medicine depends heavily on Information and Communication Technology (ICT). The environmental impact from this area is considerable, with ICT producing an estimated 2% of total global carbon emissions – about as much as the aviation industry [20]. Computers, in particular, have a limited lifetime that may only span a few years. Unless they are reused or recycled, junk computers often end up in landfill sites, thereby emitting toxins like cadmium and mercury into the soil. The health sector of course uses computers extensively for administration and patient care. Thus, there is much scope for reducing energy costs and emission from IT within the health sector by applying criteria for low-carbon manufacture, energy use and disposal of IT equipment, and through using providers that demonstrate ethical and sustainable policies. *Thin client technologies* are an example, where a computer or computer programme uses another computer (its server) to carry out traditional computing activities. By sharing the same server and using low-end computer terminals that only provide a graphical user interface, the need for individual computer terminals can be minimised. This reduces waste from equipment and lowers the total cost of ownership.

Clean technology

Harnessing renewable energy and materials for health-related products, services and processes (also called *clean technology*) is essential for reducing

> **Case study 9.2   Benefits of recycling**
>
> In the United States, more than 3000 hospitals participate in third-party medical device reprocessing, which reportedly has grown into a sizeable business generating US$ 200–250 million (£128–160 million) a year [22]. Over a period of three years, Iowa Health System, a non-profit organisation, managed to save nearly US$ 2 million (£1.3 million) and diverted over 84 000 pounds (38 100 kg) of waste from entering landfill sites through its medical device reprocessing programmes.

or even avoiding the use of natural resources and for cutting waste and emissions. Healthcare providers have many opportunities to draw on such clean technology and reduce the net quantity of resources being used (commonly defined as units of material consumption or process, for example, per in-patient bed day, per dialysis treatment, per X-ray machine or per new clinic building). Clean technologists think not just *cradle to grave*, but *cradle to cradle*, modelling processes on nature's ability to circulate nutrients in healthy and safe metabolisms [21]. Case study 9.2 illustrates how this can work in practice. Many more examples can be found in the resources listed at the end of this chapter.

The power of procurement

Procuring more sustainably is not just about buying 'greener' products and materials. Sustainable procurement in the health sector is also a way of using economic power to benefit society, the economy and the environment. This includes making decisions based on whole-life costs that include financial impact (including price and running costs), social effects (such as the impact on communities, poverty eradication, human rights and fair trade) and environmental consequences (in terms of raw materials, production and disposal) [9, 23]. The *how* and *what* of obtaining services, goods and capital in the health sector really matters. Because of the massive size of the global health sector, procuring in a sustainable way can give clear signals to manufacturers, suppliers and contractors. Case study 9.3 illustrates that this is not just wishful thinking, but that it can really work in practice.

To exert procurement power, a database of resources and suppliers with good sustainability credentials is essential. The *London Regional Public Health Group* and the *NHS Capital Investment Unit* (for the London Strategic Health Authorities), for example, have developed a simple, easy-to-use *Advisory Navigation Tool (ANT)* to provide relevant links to websites containing

---

Case study 9.3   Buying safer products and materials [24]

Kaiser Permanente, the largest not-for-profit healthcare provider in the United States, aims to identify chemicals of high concern in products and aggressively searches the market for safer alternatives. For example, to move away from powdered latex and PVC (or vinyl) examination and surgical gloves (latex can cause allergic reactions in patients and staff, and vinyl generates dioxin pollution during the manufacturing and disposal processes), this organisation decided to purchase gloves made of nitrile. Kaiser Permanente uses more than 50 million gloves each year. Resulting from its decision to buy a less harmful alternative, the entire medical glove industry was affected and responded with an increase in the supply of nitrile gloves for all glove purchasers – and lowered the cost for these.

In 2004, Kaiser Permanente was influential in developing a vinyl-free carpet that is fully recyclable and, though made from post-consumer recycled content, meets demanding performance and safety regulations. The organisation now exclusively purchases from the vendor creating this product and has installed almost a million square metres (equivalent to around 200 football pitches) of this carpet in their facilities.

---

sustainability information on topics including greener purchasing [9]. An example is the promotion of safer and 'cleaner' chemicals and anaesthetic gases [15]. Better sourcing and more effective consumption of food also has as big impact on sustainability, as explained in Chapter 6. But there is one resource that stands out because its of elemental global importance to all of us. Its supply is now increasingly threatened in many locations, and its careless sourcing and disposal can often produce considerable carbon emissions. This resource, of course, is *water*.

Using water more efficiently

Water is a precious natural resource and already scarce in many areas. More than one billion people lack access to safe and clean drinking water, and many more drink grossly contaminated water [25]. Over 3.5 billion cases of diarrhoea every year can be attributed to unsafe water and an estimated two million people, most of whom are children, die every year from diarrhoeal diseases [25]. Hydrological systems are very sensitive to climate change and even regions that are currently not affected by water shortages may suffer from drought in the coming decades. Cities such as La Paz, Bolivia, which rely on glacial melt waters for their summer supply, are particularly vulnerable. In the United Kingdom, carbon emissions from providing and disposing of household tap water account for 0.5% of the country's overall footprint. The healthcare sector, of course, consumes large quantities of water. In the case of warm or hot water, we need to remember that every litre is billed three times – for incoming fresh water, for the energy to heat the water and, finally, for the resulting sewer charges [26]. The NHS in England, for example, used a staggering 38.8 million cubic meters of water in 2007, contributing to around 26.3 million cubic metres of sewage and costing about £145 million [6]. The US Healthcare Environmental Resource Center estimates that for hospitals in the size range 133–510 beds, water use – from, for instance, water outlets, showers, toilets and laundry services – ranges from around 260 000 to 1 128 000 litres per bed per year – the equivalent of two average sized swimming pools [27].

From a sustainability perspective, using bottled water seems particularly reckless, because it carries a carbon footprint of up to 2000 times that of ordinary tap water [2]. Based on figures from the US *Pacific Institute*, the yearly consumption of bottled water in the United States in 2007 exceeded 33 billion litres and needed the energy equivalent of between 32 and 54 million barrels of oil – an amount that would be enough to provide one third of the primary US energy use [28]. As the market for bottled water continues to grow, we need to be aware of the environmental, economic and social implications. These include concerns about plastics waste, over-use of groundwater and the end costs to consumers [29]. Using bottled water also diverts municipal authorities away from the task of improving local supplies, and there is very little evidence to support the claim that bottled water is any healthier [30]. But the key item that remains is the energy used to produce and distribute bottled water in the first instance [28].

Bottled water is only part of the story. Another important first step in improving water management is to monitor and report consumption [6]. Such monitoring allows managers to respond quickly to leaks and see the impacts of water-saving interventions [1]. Smart organisations mimic natural systems by making better use of rainwater and recycling 'grey' water for non-drinking purposes. The *Sambhavna Trust Clinic* in Bhopal, India, harvests rainwater during the monsoon season, which it stores for human usage during the dryer months. The hospital also irrigates its grounds with water recycled from its waste systems [31]. The surgical wards at Gartnavel Hospital in Glasgow, UK, installed a 'knee on' tap design for surgical scrubbing, to replace the traditional elbow operated taps. By ensuring that taps are not left running needlessly, this design saves around 5.7 litres of hot water, 600 KJ of energy and around 80 grams of carbon dioxide at every scrub without compromising the quality of the procedure [32].

In the United States, the Norwood Hospital in Massachusetts consumed 29% less water in three years through water conservation, reducing consumption from 51.2 to 36.6 million gallons a year [33]. Methods to achieve this included better pump design, installing water-saving flush valves on toilets and urinals that allow better control of flow rate and volume, retrofitting lower-flow water faucets and improving refrigeration efficiency. These measures save the hospital about US$ 14 000 (£8839) every year. In the United Kingdom, a new hospital in Watford uses sustainable draining systems and rainwater harvesting/reuse methods not only to reduce the flood risk from surface water run-off but also to supply recycled rain water to Watford Football Club for watering its pitch, cleaning the stands and flushing toilets [34]. A clear win–win.

We usually only get a glimpse of the products and resources that we use. We do not know their origins or where they finally disappear to once they have reached the end of their lives. So, in the next section, we look at what happens to them and how better waste management can bring about substantial benefits.

Managing waste

In contrast to other hazardous waste, there is currently no international agreement on medical waste management, and the definition of medical waste varies from country to country [23]. Contrary to common belief, around 75–85% of hospital medical waste is similar to normal public waste. Clinical waste (as defined earlier) makes up a much smaller proportion. Approximately 3% of medical waste stems from chemical and radioactive materials and products, such as medicines, cleaning agents, laboratory chemicals and heavy metals (for example, mercury from broken thermometers), many of which can lead to harmful health and environmental effects [23]. So health services need to deal with many different forms of waste that are potentially harmful and may be difficult to manage (Figure 9.3) [35]. Issues around food waste were covered in more detail in Chapter 6.

Clinical waste in hospitals gets incinerated, but may contain up to 60% of domestic-type waste. Accordingly, the World Health Organization has identified safe and sustainable healthcare waste management as an urgent and important public health problem [36]. So what effects can health care waste have?

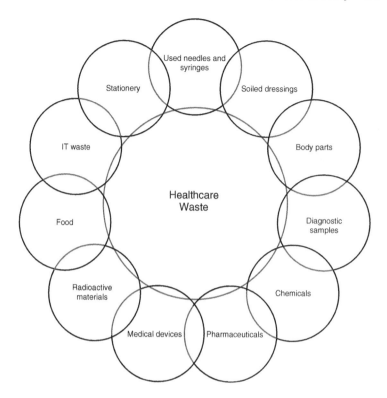

Figure 9.3 Types of healthcare waste.

Toxic effects from medical waste

The toxic and infectious parts of medical waste pose an as yet unquantified risk to environmental and human health. Findings from a systematic review suggest that over half of the world's population is at risk of health problems from toxic healthcare waste [37]. For example, hospital waste water can contain more chemicals, hazardous substances and drug-resistant pathogens than domestic sewage, and the burning of medical waste emits various hazardous compounds as well as greenhouse gases [38].

In the United Kingdom, the NHS generates one in every 100 tonnes of domestic waste arriving in landfill sites [1]. All this comes at a cost. United Kingdom figures alone show that in 2009/2010 the health service was charged with a waste bill of £83.5 million (US$134 million) [3]. Figures from the United Kingdom also demonstrate that transporting, burning and disposing

---

Case study 9.4   Making better use of organic waste [15]

The Embassy Medical Centre in Colombo, Sri Lanka, is planning to use waste from local open-air dumps to fuel the hospital's operations. This facility will collect waste through local sanitation stations near local dumps (which will also provide clean water and latrines for the local population) and meet all its energy needs through a 'waste digester' producing methane gas. The 500 000 square foot building is estimated to need 30% less energy and 40% less water to operate than other hospitals of similar size. The hospital will treat rain water to become potable and recycle grey water for landscaping and non-drinking uses. A water collection system will capture rain water during the monsoon season and store this for use in dryer seasons in the year.

---

of waste leads to about 1% (0.1 megatonnes CO_2e) of total NHS carbon emissions [39]. The case for improving waste management is indisputable. Reducing waste saves energy, costs less money and reduces the health risks connected with incineration and landfill deposition [39]. Around the world, many healthcare organisations have come up with innovative ways of rising to this challenge (Case study 9.4 gives an example).

Better waste management

Making sure that domestic waste such as paper towels is not mixed with clinical waste increases the amount of waste that can be recycled, leading directly to financial savings [40]. The *New Economics Foundation* and the *NHS Confederation* calculated that if the UK NHS segregated domestic and clinical waste correctly and recycled just 40%, the yearly carbon savings would be similar to those produced by driving an average-sized car around the equator more than 550 times [39]. To manage waste successfully, health services need appropriate facilities and procedures as well as staff who are motivated enough to change their behaviour, particularly when it comes to waste segregation. Because clinical waste is much more expensive to process, efficient segregation of clinical and non-clinical waste can save large amounts of money. The *Centre for Sustainable Healthcare* quotes one organisation saving £250 000 (US$ 395 000) per annum over several units from this intervention alone [41]. Segregation also increases recycling rates and prevents toxic waste reaching the environment. For instance, many of the plastic materials present in medical waste can be recycled. This avoids incineration which releases

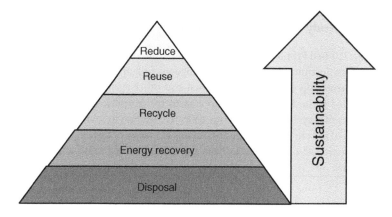

Figure 9.4 The waste hierarchy.

both greenhouse gases and atmospheric pollutants [42]. Various non-burn technologies exist to manage clinical waste safely, with autoclaving being an important alternative [36, 43]. The *waste hierarchy* (Figure 9.4) provides a useful benchmark of priorities for improving waste management. Disposal is, without doubt, the least desirable option and any strategies to manage waste better should start at the more advantageous end of the hierarchy (Case studies 9.5 and 9.6).

Avoiding waste in the first place as well as better reuse and recycling can clearly reap in both carbon and financial windfalls. To give another example, estimates for the United Kingdom forecast that recycling all the paper, cardboard, magazines and newspapers produced by the NHS could avoid up to 42 000 tons of carbon dioxide emissions every year – the equivalent of leaving 17 000 cars off the road or replacing 500 000 100-Watt incandescent light bulbs with 20-Watt energy-saving bulbs [39].

Case study 9.5   Working in collaboration [40]

Collaborative working can pay particular dividends. In the United Kingdom, the *London Procurement Programme* for example brought together more than 70 healthcare organisations to form a collaborative contract for dealing with waste. By teaming up to negotiate contracts and sharing good working practices, this collaborative has saved the NHS in London over £200 million – and continues to save over £1 million every week – while improving services and reducing clinical risk [44].

Case study 9.6   Better recycling

The 720-bed Frimley Park Hospital in the United Kingdom was the first medical institution in the United Kingdom to launch a 'Recycle Zone' in partnership with the local council and other agencies, from which recycled waste is removed at no cost to the hospital. As a result, 47 tonnes of recyclable material was collected, leading to savings of £6380 (US$ 10 214) in 2009 – while also saving 21 tonnes of carbon dioxide. It took only just over six weeks from the initial meeting to launching the scheme.

Pharmaceutical waste

Inappropriate medication disposal is widespread. This starts at home, as many people continue to flush unused medication down the toilet or throw it in the household bin – a harmful disposal practice that, as mentioned earlier, has led to trace amounts of pharmaceutical waste entering groundwater and soil. Unfortunately, regulations for pharmaceutical disposal still vary between countries. In settings where pharmaceuticals are heavily used, health services can have a major impact on minimising pharmaceutical waste by advocating better prescribing and patient information, and by better recycling (Case studies 9.7 and 9.8).

Case study 9.7   Recycling inhalers [45]

In 2011, Glaxo GlaxoSmithKline and the Cooperative Pharmacy launched the first respiratory inhaler recycling programme in Europe in partnership with TerraCycle UK. The project involved 40 Cooperative pharmacies across South Wales and the South East of England which piloted the programme for an initial six months. Participating pharmacies encouraged patients to drop off their inhalers at their store and TerraCycle UK recycled every element of the inhaler, which prevented a powerful greenhouse gas from the inhalers' propellant from being released into the environment. Because of its success, the project was extended to 200 other pharmacies. During the pilot phase, the project recycled 6000 inhalers, reducing carbon dioxide emissions by 35 tonnes – equivalent to driving an average sized car around the world six times.

> ### Case study 9.8   Ranking pharmaceuticals according to their environmental impact
>
> Sweden has made an important step forward by setting up a system that ranks pharmaceuticals according to their environmental impact, which allows health professionals as well as the public to make an informed choice towards less harmful medicines where a choice of treatments is available [8]. Initiated by *The Swedish Association of the Pharmaceutical Industry, LIF*, Sweden introduced for the first time a voluntary system for classifying pharmaceuticals according to their environmental impact, which can be accessed through a product information guide via the Internet. While the system does not yet cover all available pharmaceuticals, new information is continuously added.

Safer disposal of chemicals

To manage chemical waste effectively, institution-wide procedures and action plans for using and disposing of chemicals are essential. Safer alternatives for many chemicals are often available, such as thermometers and blood pressure devices that do not contain mercury, or less hazardous substances that replace PVC, glutaraldehyde and or nitrous oxide, which is a powerful greenhouse gas [43]. Replacing substances of very high concern with safer alternatives is of great importance, particularly where chemicals are carcinogenic, mutagenic or toxic for reproduction. Healthcare organisations can give a strong message to chemical manufacturers and distributors to manufacture safer products by developing and implementing policies that ask for disclosure of chemical ingredients in products and materials and by requiring all ingredients to have undergone at least basic toxicity testing.

Waste from medical devices and ICT

In the United Kingdom, the use of single-use devices has increased, leading to a significant rise in the volume of clinical waste [46]. Although reusable medical equipment made of glass, metal or rubber is often easy to clean and sterilise, single-use medical devices became more established as public awareness around HIV and, later, new-variant CJD grew. At present, most countries have their own regulations with regard to reusing medical equipment and reusing devices that are meant for single use. Where practical and

---

Case study 9.9   Recycling orthopaedic devices [48]

The *Brigham and Women's Hospital* in the United States now recycles titanium prostheses (which are, for example, used for hip joint replacements) for remanufacturing and reuse. This has led to substantial cost savings and reduction in mechanical breakdowns of trash disposal equipment. Replacing a waste shredder blade, for example, costs around US$ 30 000 (£19 200) – and titanium prostheses were a common cause of breakdowns.

---

legal, reusing medical equipment has the potential to save resources (Case study 9.9). The evidence base in this field is currently slim, but work is continuing to provide more definitive guidance [46]. The *American Medical Association* now promotes the recycling of unused and used medical equipment [47].

Health services can also recycle fully functioning but outmoded IT equipment for reuse in other parts of the world. *Aid for Hospitals Worldwide* is a charity setting an example of how this can be achieved [49]. This scheme collects redundant but usable medical equipment directly from site and reduces landfill as well as disposal costs for over 50 NHS hospitals. The charity estimates that 12 million people in 53 countries have benefited directly from the recycled equipment at a value of £2.3 million (US$ 3.7 million). Although storing and transporting larger amounts of equipment can cause logistic challenges and also lead to carbon emissions, these are negligible compared to the alternatives [49].

Managing resources for the future

As we have outlined in this chapter, the opportunities for supporting sustainable consumption are substantial. By procuring responsibly and ethically, health services have the chance to help protect natural resources, create more sustainable communities and set an important example for businesses and the public sector [23]. New strategies for better resource management are being developed all the time and, as we have demonstrated, there are many examples of good practice. To help share such knowledge, a list of useful resources is provided at the end of this chapter. Health services can – and must – play an important role in moving toward a system where no more natural resources are being used than can be replenished.

All clinical care demands natural and fiscal resources, and we have looked in previous chapters at how we can reduce such costs whilst maintaining and improving the quality of what we do. There is one domain of practice that is especially resource intensive and which has much to teach us about what lies at the core of sustainable healthcare: care at the end of life. Because of the enormity of the challenges that this part of medical care poses, and because of the opportunities that health services have to improve the *quality of life* of those who are terminally ill rather than prolonging it artificially and perhaps unnecessarily, we devote the next chapter to this topic.

Key actions

Procurement

- Consider the most appropriate stock levels, so that supply is appropriate but items do not get past their 'use by' dates unused.
- Team up with other healthcare partners to increase buying power for ethically produced and sustainable products.
- Follow ethical procurement guidance (such as from the *British Medical Association*) [19].
- Evaluate ways of reusing or recycling items before new ones are ordered.
- Take into account the whole lifecycle cost of any purchase, including financial, ethical and social and environmental impacts (such as carbon emissions, waste, toxicity, resource implications from raw materials used in the production etc.).
- Ask suppliers to demonstrate their methods for sustainable development and reducing carbon emissions.
- Support local manufacturers and vendors who produce third party certified sustainable products and follow ethical and sustainable practices where possible
- Advocate for products which generate minimum (or even zero) waste, are long-life, are less disposable, contain a minimum of hazardous raw materials and use less packaging.

Water management

- Only wash full loads of dishes and laundry.
- Use short showers instead of baths, and share baths.
- Avoid buying bottled water.

- Turn off the tap when brushing teeth.
- Measure water use and feed the amounts of water used back to people and teams, and track changes over time.
- Eliminate the use of bottled water in your organisation if high quality tap water is available.
- Locate and fix leaking appliances and reduce unnecessary flow in kitchens, bathrooms and laboratories and on hospital wards.
- Avoid unnecessary ground irrigation.
- Install efficient low-flush or dual flush volume toilet cisterns.
- Install flow reducers and aerators on showers and automatic shut-off valves or motion sensor-activated taps where appropriate.
- Replace any appliances or pieces of equipment with water-saving models.
- Install pressure-reducing valves where appropriate.
- Investigate sources of used or rain water.
- Plant drought resistant plants on your premises to minimise the need for irrigation.
- Look for opportunities to recycle water on site (for example, recycling water from dialysis machines or sterilisers).
- Switch to all-digital imaging technology where possible, which saves water and reduces toxic chemical residue.
- Implement policies to measure and monitor water costs and consumption, and report these in regular interval to patients, staff and the wider public.
- Increase awareness of the importance of responsible water use conservation and educate staff, patients and visitors.

Medicines management (Data from [43])

- Organise centralised pharmaceutical waste collections.
- Avoid over-procurement and maintain strict control of stocks (preferably using those items that are coming up to their expiry date).
- Inform patients about safe disposal of expired or unused medicines and encourage them to return unused medication to the dispensing pharmacy.
- Recycle inhalers.
- Prescribe small initial quantities for new prescriptions and dispense only the amount needed.
- Implement 'low stock' policies in pharmacies to reduce the amount of medicines that go out of date before being dispensed.

- Develop training programmes for prescribers around optimal prescribing practices.
- Advocate for manufacturers (who are familiar with the exact chemical composition of their products) to take back unused stock [50].
- In low-income countries, encapsulating drugs or making them inert by mixing them with concrete are cheap and effective approaches before disposal in landfill.

Waste

- Segregate waste as appropriate and recycle non-hazardous products and materials.
- Develop and introduce a broad programme to reduce waste.
- Bring in non-burn technology and avoid incineration where practical and possible.
- Press public authorities to build and maintain secure landfill sites to manage non-recyclable waste that has been adequately treated.
- Avoid purchasing toxic materials such as PVC, mercury and unnecessary disposable products.
- Establish a waste management committee in your organisation with a dedicated budget.
- Reduce the volume and toxicity of waste through implementing environmentally sound waste management and disposal options.
- Make sure staff in your organisation are trained in managing waste safely and effectively.
- Reduce overall waste to landfill, and recycle and compost where practical.
- Reduce hazardous waste and waste from clinical areas.
- Avoid or eliminate medical waste incineration.
- Implement strategies to minimise waste and reuse or recycle where possible.
- Comply with sustainability legislation.
- Press public authorities to build and maintain secure landfill sites to manage non-recyclable waste that has been adequately treated.

Further reading and information

Various tools, guidance documents and frameworks exist to help organisations procure better and tackle waste and water issues. A selection of useful websites is shown in Box 9.1.

Box 9.1   Sources of further information

- British Medical Association, *Ethical Procurement for Health*, http://www.bma.org.uk/international/international_development /fairtrade/ethicalprocurehealthworkbook.jsp
- Department for Environment, Food and Rural Affairs (DEFRA), www.defra.gov.uk
- Global Green and Healthy Hospitals Network, www.greenhospitals.net
- Healthcare Without Harm, www.noharm.org
- Healthier Hospitals Initiative, www.healthierhospitals.org
- Practice Greenhealth, http://practicegreenhealth.org
- The Caroline Walker Trust, www.cwt.org.uk
- UK Sustainable Development Unit, www.sdu.nhs.uk (*Procuring for Carbon Reduction (P4CR)* document, jointly produced with the Department of Health).

References

1. N.H.S. Sustainable Development Unit (2009) Saving Carbon, Improving Health: Carbon Reduction Strategy for England. NHS Sustainable Development Unit, Cambridge.
2. Berners-Lee, M. (2010) *How Bad Are Bananas?: The carbon footprint of everything*. Profile Books, London.
3. NHS Information Centre – Hospital Estates and Facilities Statistics [Internet]. http://www.hefs.ic.nhs.uk/ReportFilterConfirm.asp?FilterOpen=&Year=2009% 2F2010&Level=T&Section=S11&SHA=&Org_Type=&Foundation=&Site_ Type=&PFI=&getReport=Get+Report [accessed 13 September 2011].
4. NHS National Innovation Centre – The Waste-Watcher Toolkit [Internet]. http://showcase.nic.nhs.uk/ShowcaseDetails.aspx?id=9 [accessed 7 November 2011].
5. PricewaterhouseCoopers LLP (2009) Top 10 health industry issues in 2010: PwC [Internet]. http://www.pwc.com/us/en/healthcare/publications/top-ten-health -industry-issues-in-2010.jhtml [accessed 31 October 2011].
6. UK Department of Health (2009). Health technical memorandum. The Stationery Office, London.
7. UK Sustainable Development Unit (2008, updated 2009) Carbon Emissions Carbon Footprinting Report [Internet]. http://www.sdu.nhs.uk/documents /publications/1263313924_jgyW_nhs_england_carbon_emissions_carbon_ footprinting_r.pdf [accessed June 2011].
8. FASS.se – Startsida [Internet]. http://www.fass.se/LIF/home/index.jsp [accessed 1 November 2011].

9. National Institute for Health and Clinical Excellence (2005) Making the case for sustainable procurement: the NHS as a good corporate citizen [Internet]. http://www.nice.org.uk/niceMedia/docs/Making_the_case-Procurement.pdf [accessed 13 September 2011].

10. Doerr-MacEwen, N.A. and Haight, M.E. (2006) Expert Stakeholders' Views on the Management of Human Pharmaceuticals in the Environment. *Environmental Management*, 38, 853–866.

11. AstraZeneca – Ecopharmacovigilance [Internet]. http://www.astrazeneca.com /environmental-product-stewardship/Ecopharmacovigilance [accessed 2 March 2012].

12. Collaborative on Health and the Environment–CHE Toxicant and Disease Database [Internet]. http://www.healthandenvironment.org/tddb [accessed 2 November 2011].

13. Prüss-Ustün, A., Vickers, C., Haefliger, P. and Bertollini, R. (2011) Knowns and unknowns on burden of disease due to chemicals: a systematic review. *Environmental Health*, 10, 9.

14. WHO (2010) Strategic Approach to International Chemicals Management (SAICM): Health Sector Focus [Internet]. http://www.who.int/ipcs/saicm/saicm_ health/en/index.html [accessed 2 November 2011].

15. World Health Organization and Healthcare Without Harm. (2009) Healthy hospitals, healthy planet, healthy people: Addressing climate change in healthcare settings [Internet]. http://www.who.int/globalchange/publications/healthcare_ settings/en/index.html [accessed 2 August 2011].

16. UK Department of Health (2010) New study on medicine waste [Internet]. http://www.dh.gov.uk/en/Aboutus/Features/DH_122051 [accessed 18 September 2011].

17. UK Department of Health (2011) Making best use of medicines: Report of a Department of Health roundtable event hosted by The King's Fund [Internet]. http://www.dh.gov.uk/en/Publicationsandstatistics/Publications /PublicationsPolicyAndGuidance/DH_128283 [accessed 18 September 2011].

18. Kalorama Information (2011) Medical Device Revenue to Top $300 Billion This Year [Internet]. http://www.kaloramainformation.com/about/release.asp?id= 1826 [accessed 1 November 2011].

19. The British Medical Association – Ethical Procurement for Health [Internet]. http://www.bma.org.uk/international/international_development/fairtrade /ethicalprocurehealthworkbook.jsp [accessed 1 November 2011].

20. EcoFriend (2007) Computers emit as much carbon dioxide as aviation [Internet]. http://www.ecofriend.com/entry/computers-emit-as-much-carbon-dioxide-as- aviation/ [accessed 18 September 2011].

21. Braungart, M. and McDonough, W. (2009) *Cradle to Cradle*. Vintage Books.

22. Razor, T. (2010) Recycling boosts Iowa Health's bottom line [Internet]. http:// www.ihs.org/body.cfm?id=67&Action=detail&ref=187 [accessed 4 December 2011].

23. Department for Environment, Food and Rural Affairs (2006) Procuring the future [Internet]. http://www.defra.gov.uk/publications/files/pb11710- procuring-the-future-060607.pdf [accessed 12 September 2011].

24. Kaiser Permanente – Case Study: Using Safer Chemicals in Products Supports Preventive Health Care [Internet]. http://www.saferchemicals.org/resources /business/kaiser-permanente.html [accessed 2 March 2012].

25. WHO (2007) Combating waterborne disease at the household level [Internet]. http://www.who.int/household_water/advocacy/combating_disease/en/index .html [accessed 3 November 2011].

26. ENERGY STAR (2005) Saving Water Counts in Energy Efficiency: [Internet]. http://www.energystar.gov/index.cfm?c=healthcare.ashe_sept_oct_2005 [accessed 20 April 2012].

27. Healthcare Environmental Resource Center (HERC) – Facilities Management: Water Conservation [Internet]. http://www.hercenter.org/facilitiesandgrounds /waterconserve.cfm [accessed 31 October 2011].

28. Gleick, P.H. and Cooley, H.S. (2009) Energy implications of bottled water. *Environmental Research Letters*. [Internet] http://www.mwra.state.ma.us/04water /html/bullet1.htm, 014009.

29. Wagner, M. and Oehlmann, J. (2011) Endocrine disruptors in bottled mineral water: estrogenic activity in the E-Screen. *Journal of Steroid Biochemistry and Molecular Biology* **127** (1–2), 128–135.

30. McCartney, M. (2011)Waterlogged? *British Medical Journal*, **343** (2), d4280.

31. Guenther, R. and Vittori, G. (2008) *Sustainable healthcare architecture.* John Wiley and Sons Ltd, Chichester.

32. Somner, J.E.A., Stone, N., Koukkoulli, A., Scott, K.M., Field, A.R. and Zygmunt, J. (2008) Surgical scrubbing: can we clean up our carbon footprints by washing our hands? *Journal of Hospital Infection*, **70**, 212–215.

33. Massachusetts Water Resources Authority (MWRA) – Water Use Case Study: Norwood Hospital [Internet]. http://www.mwra.state.ma.us/04water/html /bullet1.htm [accessed 18 September 2011].

34. Watford Health Campus – Sustainability [Internet]. http://www .watfordhealthcampus.info/the-project/masterplan/environment/sustainability [accessed 7 November 2011].

35. WHO – Medical waste [Internet]. http://www.who.int/topics/medical_waste/en/ [accessed 16 September 2011].

36. WHO (2007) WHO core principles for achieving safe and sustainable management of health-care waste [Internet]. http://www.who.int/water_sanitation_health /medicalwaste/hcwprinciples/en/index.html [accessed 3 November 2011].

37. Harhay, M.O., Halpern, S.D., Harhay, J.S. and Olliaro, P.L. (2009) Health care waste management: a neglected and growing public health problem worldwide. *Tropical Medicine & International Health*, **14**, 1414–1417.

38. Health Care Without Harm (2011) UN Human Rights Report Calls for An End to Medical Waste Incineration [Internet]. http://www.noharm.org/global/news_ hcwh/2011/sep/hcwh2011-09-14.php [accessed 3 November 2011].

39. NHS Confederation, (2007) Taking the temperature: towards an NHS response to global warming. The NHS Confederation, London.

40. London Procurement Programme – Waste management [Internet]. http://www .lpp.nhs.uk/page.asp?fldArea=2&fldMenu=3&fldSubMenu=1&fldKey=72 [accessed 17 September 2011].

41. Centre for Sustainable Healthcare – Cost Benefits of SAP [Internet]. http://
sap.greenerhealthcare.org/benefits/cost-benefits [accessed 6 March 2012].

42. UK Department of Health (2011) Safe management of healthcare waste
[Internet]. http://www.dh.gov.uk/en/Publicationsandstatistics/Publications
/PublicationsPolicyAndGuidance/DH_126345 [accessed 17 September 2011].

43. Health Care Without Harm (2011) Launches Global Environmental Health
Agenda for Hospitals [Internet]. http://www.noharm.org/global/news_hcwh
/2011/oct/hcwh2011-10-13.php [accessed 3 November 2011].

44. London Procurement Programme – Our achievements [Internet]. http://www.
lpp.nhs.uk/page.asp?fldArea=1&fldMenu=2&fldSubMenu=0&fldKey=28
[accessed 17 September 2011].

45. Centre for Sustainable Healthcare (2012) Innovative Inhaler Recycling
Project Expanded [Internet].http://sustainablehealthcare.org.uk/blog/2012/01
/innovative-inhaler-recycling-project-expanded-0 [accessed 6 March 2012].

46. Sustainable Operating Theatres [Internet]. http://sustainablehealthcare.org.uk
/sustainable-operating-theatres/feed [accessed 31 October 2011].

47. American Medical Association – Medical Supply Recycling Programs [Internet].
http://www.ama-assn.org/ama/pub/about-ama/our-people/member-groups-
sections/medical-student-section/community-service/medical-supply-recycling-
programs.page [accessed 31 October 2011].

48. BWH Bulletin (2007) Operation Recycle Underway in OR [Internet].
http://www.brighamandwomens.org/about_bwh/publicaffairs/news/publications
/DisplayBulletin.aspx?articleid=3868 [accessed 2 March 2012].

49. Aid to Hospitals Worldwide (Recycling medical equipment to save lives ...)
(Home) [Internet]. http://www.a2hw.org.uk/ [accessed 6 March 2012].

50. WHO (1999) Guidelines for Safe Disposal of Unwanted Pharmaceuticals
in and after Emergencies [Internet]. http://apps.who.int/medicinedocs/en/d
/Jwhozip51e/ [accessed 1 November 2011].

Chapter 10 **The Green Death**

'It is the duty of a doctor to prolong life. It is not his duty to prolong death.'

(attributed to Sir Thomas Horder [1871–1955], Physician)

In this chapter

- Death and sustainability
- The costs of death and dying
- Towards a greener death

Our way of death has a lot to teach us about our way of life. Though death, like taxation, is one of life's few certainties, our relationship to it in the developed world has become remote. It is not something that usually carries us off in the prime of life but mostly something that closes upon us when we are old and infirm. Most people have little direct experience of the dead body, often whisked away to the funeral parlour, maybe never to be seen again – in contrast to poorer countries, where death is a more palpable companion. Health professionals are unusual in having, through their work and training, more intimate relations with the dying process than the average citizen. They therefore have the potential to guide people through the labyrinth of choices that surround death, bringing insight into what for most remains an unvoiced and difficult topic. Dying is not only something intimate; death and its approaches are a major strand of the healthcare enterprise, with far-reaching sustainability implications. This chapter examines the human, fiscal and environmental costs of the period leading up to death and of our care for the body after death. It then explores a range of ways in which health professionals can participate in a greener, and better, way of death.

Sustainable Healthcare, First Edition. Knut Schroeder, Trevor Thompson, Kathleen Frith and David Pencheon.
© 2013 John Wiley & Sons, Ltd. Published 2013 by John Wiley & Sons, Ltd.

Death and sustainability

Death is a stark reminder of the finite, in a culture where we have, erroneously, come to think of resources as inexhaustible and continued growth as inevitable. Who ever heard a politician say something like 'I am happy to report that in line with its natural tendency to oscillate, the economy shrank a bit this year'? The myth of continual growth shows parallels to the myth of eternal youth. According to Reuters, United States' citizens spent US$ 10 billion ($6.4 billion) on plastic surgery in 2009, much of which is seeking to escape the inescapable truth of aging [1]. Whilst some of our most important resources, like compassion, are perfectly renewable, most things come in cycles that require involution as well as growth. So to think sustainably is to think cyclically, which includes accepting the inevitability of death – including our own. By accepting death we can make of it something which we can experience in its fullness, as appeared to have been the case with a ceremony recorded in the book 'After Life' (Box 10.1).

Not too soon though. Medical technology keeps death at bay. In our lectures we ask for a show of hands of those who think that without medical inventions they would now be dead (excluding preventative measures). A third of students perceive this to be the case. Naturally, this is something to celebrate. Anyone who has been scooped up by an ambulance after a nasty accident or wept as their child was saved from a catastrophic infection will be hard to convince that *less* healthcare might be *better* healthcare. But it is a curious paradox that *less* might in fact mean *more*, particularly, as we shall

Box 10.1   Death and dying as a positive experience

'My mum's funeral, whilst in accordance with her wishes, was not for her benefit. It was for the benefit of us left behind, an opportunity for us to say our goodbyes, make our peace, to reflect and consider. Mum chose a wonderful spot in a private area overlooking the hills and under a large shady oak tree. Her choosing of a place rather than being allocated an anonymous plot made it personal and underlined that she had faced up to and accepted her death. Sun and rain alternated, all things grow, die and regenerate. People cried, people hugged, people even smiled. My mother's love of nature, of life, came through in her choice of funeral. It turned what could have been a sterile necessity of an occasion into a life affirming event.'

Quotation from Ian Ross-Bain in After Life (edited by Stephanie Weinrich) [2]

see, at the end of life. This paradox is underpinned by a complicated tension between the inevitability of death and our recent capacities for sustaining biological life – a tension that exacts a heavy toll on our fragile systems.

Heroic interventions

This tension centres on the vexed distinction between what is medically possible and what is clinically appropriate. Medical interventions are easy to start, but difficult to withdraw once initiated. Patients and families seem to invite heroic intervention while at the same time they may 'fear losing their lives to the medical system' [3]. The Boston surgeon Atul Gawande shares several anecdotes of over-intervention in his 2010 *New Yorker* article, in which he champions the role of hospice care in the face of boundless medicalisation (Box 10.2) [4]. What drives the health professions to these potentially futile end-of-life interventions, such as aggressive chemotherapy

---

Box 10.2 Cases cited in a *New Yorker* article by Atul Gawande [4]

Recently, while seeing a patient in an intensive care unit (ICU) at my hospital, I stopped to talk with the critical care physician on duty, someone I'd known since college. 'I'm running a warehouse for the dying', she said bleakly. Out of the ten patients in her unit, she said, only two were likely to leave the hospital for any length of time. More typical was an almost eighty-year-old woman at the end of her life, with irreversible congestive heart failure, who was in the ICU for the second time in three weeks, drugged to oblivion and tubed in most natural orifices and a few artificial ones. Or the seventy-year-old with a cancer that had metastasised to her lungs and bone, and a fungal pneumonia that arises only in the final phase of the illness. She had chosen to forgo treatment, but her oncologist pushed her to change her mind, and she was put on a ventilator and antibiotics. Another woman, in her eighties, with end-stage respiratory and kidney failure, had been in the unit for two weeks. Her husband had died after a long illness, with a feeding tube and a tracheotomy, and she had mentioned that she did not want to die that way. But her children could not let her go and asked to proceed with the placement of various devices: a permanent tracheotomy, a feeding tube and a dialysis catheter. So now she just lay there tethered to her pumps, drifting in and out of consciousness.

in incurable cancer? We know that fear of litigation prompts investigations and procedures [5], and that relatives can push for intensive care, with perhaps unrealistic expectation of its likely benefit. Societal expectations of technology are also influenced by valiant portrayals in medical television dramas [6]. This drive for biological life at the expense of quality of life indicates a universal discomfort with the facts of death to which doctors are not immune. In a Chicago hospice setting, the terminal prognoses offered by 343 physicians were compared with actual survival in 468 individual cases. In 63% of occasions the physicians overestimated survival. The ratio of the mean *predicted* survival period to the mean of *actual* survival was 5.3 [7]. This would suggest that even experienced physicians struggle to convey the final realities of death – a certainty that every other part of their training has been designed to avert. Whilst some might approve of such optimism, others might see it as something that deprives the patient of an opportunity to make timely preparations, both inwardly and practically.

The different costs of care

The human cost of a besieged hospital death can be high, both for the patient and their loved ones, as illustrated in case vignettes from the Gawande article cited in Box 10.2. An estimated 75% of Americans die in hospital, and 20% in intensive care beds, likely sedated and possibly restrained to prevent tubes being tugged out. According to the *Cicely Saunders Foundation*, the figure for hospital deaths was 53% in the United Kingdom in 2010, with only 21% dying at home [8]. This same report provides survey evidence that 89% of persons *wished* to die at home or in a hospice.

From a systems perspective, the fiscal and carbon costs of this mismatch are equally concerning. Of course, health needs are greater in the last year of life, so expenditure would be expected to rise in parallel. But the extent of spending at the end is concerning. For instance, more than 30% of the United States' Medicaid budget is consumed in the last year of life. If that spending was necessary, we would expect levels of spending to be consistent within different regions of a country. But even within the United States, there are startling differences [9]. Research from the *Dartmouth Atlas Project* shows that people dying in Miami might have 46 specialist appointments in the last six months of their lives, spend six days in an intensive care unit and stand a 27% chance of dying in one, at a total average cost of around US$ 23 000 (£14 500) [10]. But anyone spending those same last six months in Portland, Oregon, will go to the doctor 18 times, spend one day in intensive care and stand a 13% chance of dying there at a total average cost of US$ 14 000 (£8800). There is no evidence to suggest that those dying at greater cost in Florida have a better experience. In fact, since palliative care services are well developed in Oregon, the opposite might be true (the State is rated sixth in the United States by the Centre to Advance Palliative care) [11]. Thus, it seems fair to conclude that financial and physical resources may at times be systemically squandered in care at the end of life.

The carbon costs of dying

We currently lack precise data on the carbon costs of medical care at the end of life. One assumption would be to consider carbon costs proportional to fiscal costs. Obviously, some proportionality exists, but the nature of end-of-life care brings in some systematic bias. For instance, once someone is considered terminally ill, care is mainly supportive, with a focus on symptom control rather than heroic intervention, assuming palliative care services are in place. With a cancer diagnosis, such palliative care is likely to be less carbon intensive than 'active treatment', though with other diagnoses such as heart failure there is no such clear transition to a palliative phase. What active treatment entails varies hugely by locale. For instance, Gawande quotes an average spend of US$ 63 000 (£39 700) during the last six months of life for an incurable breast cancer in the United States. No formal carbon audit of such care has yet been undertaken. The UK NHS Sustainable Development Unit has provided a breakdown of the carbon costs for NHS England as a whole, which gives us some indicative figures. Surprisingly, three fifths of the NHS's carbon footprint stem from procurement. Of this, half is attributable to pharmaceuticals and medical equipment, with pharmaceuticals contributing a fifth of the total for NHS England [12]. Further light is shed by a carbon audit of a UK renal service, showing that 35% of the overall renal service footprint arose from pharmaceuticals [13]. Thus, medication is likely to contribute considerably to the carbon cost of end-of-life care.

The costs after death

We have dealt so far with the medical costs of dying. A patient's death may be the 'end of the spend' for the healthcare system but also the start of another big set of costs, both fiscal and environmental. When someone dies, typical costs include body removal and preparation, coffin purchase, notice payments, hearse and limousine hire, church service fees, burial or cremation expenses, catering arrangements and any permanent memorial. For the United Kingdom cost estimates vary but hover at around £6000 (US$ 9470). They are higher in the United States, with average figures of around US$ 12 000 (£7603). Most of this expenditure is mediated by funeral directors who offer an invaluable service for relatives coping with the emotional and practical effects of bereavement.

But the bereaved can also be vulnerable to exploitation by commercial forces. The book *Grave Matters* by Mark Harris investigates the practices of the US funeral industry and reveals how such high levels of expenditure can build up [14]. The bereaved family is typically presented with funeral 'packages' or can choose options from a 'General Price List'. Embalming, for instance, will cost US$ 825 (£520), and some companies will not permit viewing of the dead body without it. The viable alternative of refrigeration is not usually mentioned. The family will be shown the company's range of caskets, including those made of bronze or copper, which can be made impervious to water and cost US$ 4000–10 000 (£2535–6336). A message comes across that the bereaved can signal their love of the deceased through the quality and quantity of the provision they make for the funeral. Especially when a death is unexpected, the bereaved may lack the resources to question what is being proposed, and to do so might even seem disrespectful. Though there are benefits in having 'everything taken care of', coming generations may increasingly seek to make choices more fitting with the values of the deceased (for example through *Advanced Directives*, which we cover later in this chapter).

Costing cremation

Considering the environmental costs of death and dying helps us to gain a systems-based understanding of what we do with our dead. 70% of persons are cremated after death in the United Kingdom, about half that figure in the United States. Cheaper than burial, this has the immediate appeal of saving space, as our major urban centres are currently running out of room. 'Double burial' on sites of old graves is now essential in space-strapped Tokyo and in London, where over 15 000 people are laid to rest in the ground every year. Estimates of the carbon costs of cremation are hard to secure, as they depend on many variables, including the size of the dead person, coffin materials and whether persons are cremated singly or in batches [15]. Cremation works at very high temperatures (more than 1000°C) and takes over two hours. One estimate puts the energy cost at 730 kWh (or 1.3 British Thermal Units, BTU, of gas per hour), which is substantial given that the average US citizen uses 8000 kWh of electricity in a year [16]. In addition to carbon emissions, cremation emits other contaminants, including mercury from dental fillings. In the United Kingdom, crematoriums are responsible for 16% of all mercury emissions, though the industry is working toward a 50% reduction by 2012 [17]. The mercury content of human remains is set to increase as people die having had more restorative dentistry – a clear example of a failure to think systemically.

The bad news about burial

Burial avoids such direct energy consumption, but some burial practices are much greener than others. Though cremation is an ancient and widespread practice, the return of the body's composition to the earth feels, to some, like a more 'natural' option. Its greenness depends on what gets buried, because this is often much more than just the body. In many countries the practice of embalming is commonplace. Embalming substances are used to preserve the body in the period up to burial (or cremation) so that it looks better in terms of shape and colour. Combined with grooming practices, this is seen as an important aide in the grieving process. Embalming involves replacing body fluids with a formaldehyde solution. Eva Collins, of the University of Waikato, New Zealand, quotes the Unites States' 22 500 cemeteries as burying more than three million litres of embalming fluid per annum [18]. Formaldehyde is classed as a carcinogen by the National Toxicity Program in the Unites States, though the toxicity of buried formaldehyde is uncertain, as it is metabolised in soils. In the Unites States it is common practice to bury the dead in hardwood coffins within steel-reinforced concrete vaults, further delaying the decomposition of the body. Collins quotes the annual use of 1.5 million tonnes of reinforced concrete and nearly 13 000 tonnes of steel for vaults, as well as more than 10 million metres of hardwood board for coffins (much of it tropical). The investment of so many resources in the preservation of the dead seems like an extension of our valiant efforts to preserve the living, and reminiscent of the practices of ancient cultures such as the Egyptians. Even the more typical burial in a wooden coffin 'six feet under' places the body at a depth where the soil is relatively lifeless and a return to the elements slow.

Toward a greener death

So far we have raised some serious concerns about our way of death and dying. What can we do to make our practices better for people and planet? As with many sustainability issues, the answer lies between what we can do personally, what we can do as health professionals and how best practice can be reflected in organisational and national policies. As any clinician knows, once technological interventions have been initiated it can very difficult to overturn them. And so a key concept in the Green Death is that of *preparation*. The preparation needed is both inward and outward and concerns both the dying process and what to do after the time of death. There are interesting analogies here with birth. Whilst some will eschew the idea of the 'birth plan' for such a notoriously unpredictable life event, few would argue that it is not a good idea to prepare for the birth of a child. Things to consider include having a bag with the necessary stuff ready for the start of labour, helping existing children prepare emotionally, talking to friends and relatives about their experiences, reading books on what to expect and maybe visiting a labour ward. We would argue that just the same level of interest could be applied to death and dying. This could be a very solemn undertaking but also a source of comfort, insight and a certain amount of morbid humour. A leading voice in this field in the United Kingdom is the Natural Death Centre (www.naturaldeath.org.uk); its *Natural Death Handbook* is a practically orientated text that every United Kingdom practitioner should have at hand [19]. Its cultural mission could be summarised as an attempt to make death an end in itself (and so perhaps something to be celebrated) rather than just the end of the self (and therefore something to be feared and shunned).

Embracing death

We do not feel qualified to offer advice on how health workers should prepare inwardly for their own death but, nevertheless, this is a critical aspect of the *Green Death*. Why? Because if health professionals are unprepared, then that lack of preparedness is going to be projected onto their care of others, together with the negative consequences we have already examined [20]. In lacking preparedness, health professionals are no different to the rest of society but their attitude to death has much more wide-ranging effects. In systems terms, death is an example, like atmospheric gases, of a 'hidden part'. Healthy and resilient systems embrace their parts and are in communication with them. Religious teachers from all traditions voice respect for death as a teacher, a fact that focuses us on the present and the possibilities of preparation. This is a perspective that is particularly alive in the Tibetan Buddhist tradition:

> Normally we do not like to think about death.
> We would rather think about life.
> Why reflect on death?
> When you start preparing for death you soon realize
> that you must look into your life now . . .
> and come to face the truth of your self.
> Death is like a mirror
> in which the true meaning of life
> is reflected.
>
> *(Sogyal Rinpoche)*

Talking about death

Patients benefit hugely from carers who have the poise to initiate sensitive discussions around death and dying – yet so often they do not occur. For instance, in one questionnaire study of 152 outpatients, 68% wanted to discuss end-of-life care decisions with their physician, though only 6% had actually done so [21]. Studies of patients following such discussions have failed to demonstrate psychological harm [22]. Awareness of these problems led the *UK's National Council for Palliative Care* to set up the *Dying Matters Coalition*. Its website (www.dyingmatters.org) is highly recommended. It has a membership of over 14 000 persons and links to educational offerings for health professionals. Aspects that might be good to address in end-of-life care discussions can be found in Box 10.3.

It is good to initiate discussions about end-of-life issues early in the trajectory of a progressive life-limiting illness. Whereas before such discussions arose when patients became 'terminal', current best practice suggests that planning discussions should be triggered by a negative answer to the question 'would you be surprised if this patient died within the next 6–12 months' [23]? Whilst rapid and progressive decline is often seen in cancer, deterioration in conditions such as chronic obstructive pulmonary disease (COPD) or heart failure can be more remitting and unpredictable, which is a challenge and part of the reason why palliative care in such conditions is less developed.

Advanced planning

Books such as the *Natural Death Handbook* give advice around the practical issues of preparing for death [19]. Important issues to consider as part of this

Box 10.3 Examples of content for end-of-life care discussions

- Spiritual and religious beliefs.
- Persons to be called upon to help with decision making.
- Thoughts about place of death.
- Thoughts on different types of interventions at the end of life.
- Personal ways of doing things.
- Special concerns – for example the care of pets.
- Fears about what might happen.

process include writing a will (60% of persons in the United Kingdom die intestate), recording messages to loved ones, putting financial affairs in order, nominating people to act on the person's behalf and making funeral plans. We focus here on aspects of preparation that have direct implications for health professionals and the Green Death. *Advanced Directives* (also known as *Living Wills*) are written statements made at a time when a person is of sound mind, to indicate that individual's preferences with respect to medical treatment should they become unable for medical reasons to express them directly [24]. The legal status of these documents varies from country to country, and their legality has never been tested in the English courts. Whilst a person could state a preference for having as much life-sustaining care as medically possible, such requests would not be legally binding. Advanced Directives are mainly about what people *do not* want to receive, and as such represent another possible virtuous cycle. By limiting potentially futile treatments, individuals benefit themselves and the environment.

There is no set structure for an Advanced Directive. Typically it includes a statement of the sorts of situations that the Advanced Directive would apply to, for instance a severe stroke or the development of dementia. It then specifies the types of intervention that the person would and would not accept in that situation. It also tends to contain details of persons who could help interpret the Advanced Directive, and when and how it will be reviewed. The ethical issues associated with Advanced Directives are extremely complex. For instance, how do we judge that a given condition is definitely irreversible? How do we know that a critically ill and non-communicative self would have the same views and values as the self that wrote the Advanced Directive in the past? Despite these problems, we view the Advanced Directive as a useful part of end-of-life-care planning, not least because the creation of the document gives the person, their family and their professional carers an excellent opportunity to discuss these vital issues prior to their actual emergence. Alternatively, a statement of the person's general values may be a better aid to care planning than a legalistic Advance Directive [25].

Health professionals who make their own Living Wills will have a head start when it comes to negotiating those of patients. If a patient presents one, this should never simply be filed, as this would waste the opportunity for an important discussion that should include family members and the stated 'health care proxy'. There is a good case for the proxy not being a close family member, as emotional bonds may interfere with interpretation. Professionals should guard against imposing their values on those of the patient, but neither should they relinquish their clinical judgement. Might an overly forthright statement signal an underlying depression for instance?

And has the patient thought through complexities such as the *palliative* role of modalities like radiotherapy and surgery? As in so many aspects of healthcare, the *partnership* model is best. Advanced Directives should be carefully stored and flagged in clinical notes, so that they are at hand at the time when important decisions need to be made. This is particularly important when deputising services are employed and on first admission to hospital.

A more specific aspect of end-of-life care planning is the '*do not resuscitate*' or 'DNR' order, used to establish whether or not people should receive cardio-pulmonary resuscitation when their heart stops beating or they stop breathing. The quality of life and the sustainability implications of such discussions are considerable, as a DNR decision can avoid inappropriate admissions to hospital and intensive care units [25]. Because the phrase 'do not resuscitate' implies that something is being withheld, orders are now often being renamed as '*allow natural death*' (AND), emphasising in a positive way what is being done rather than what is being held back [26].

The impact of advanced planning

Does advance care planning actually impact on the level of intervention at the end of life? And is there a cost in terms of longevity? In fiscal, carbon and human terms we know that hospital admissions are costly for patients at the end of their lives. Studies have shown that highly integrated primary care systems, where physicians look to the care of individually known patients, hospital admission rates are much lower (by a third in one study) [27]. In a multicentre study of 332 patients, 37.0% reported having end-of-life discussions at baseline [28]. Those who had such discussions experienced lower rates of ventilation, resuscitation and ICU admission. More aggressive medical care (for example mechanical ventilation) was associated with worse patient quality of life and higher risk of major depressive disorder in bereaved caregivers. This study did not measure fiscal and carbon costs, but with less intensive care it is likely that these will be proportionately reduced. A cluster randomised controlled trial conducted in Canadian nursing homes studied the cost implications of a programme encouraging advanced directives [29]. Healthcare use was studied over an 18-month period in matched nursing homes. Intervention nursing homes reported fewer hospitalisations per resident and less resource use. The average total cost per patient was C\$ 3490 (US\$ 3516 or £2228) compared to C\$ 5239 (US\$ 5279 or £3345) in control nursing homes. The proportion of deaths in both comparison groups was similar, as were the scores of patient satisfaction. Again, carbon savings can be inferred. These data suggest a virtuous cycle, in which planning issues around death and dying benefits both people and planet.

The dementia question

It would be disingenuous to skirt round the sustainability implications of dementia. Increasingly large numbers of people in our population live with *severe* dementia and depend on others for their daily survival but are, arguably, unable to partake meaningfully in social life. In 2008 the cost of dementia care in the European Union was estimated at 160 billion Euros (counting both direct and informal costs) [30]. Many people do not wish to live a drawn out existence with severe dementia. They do not wish to see their personal savings and public resources expended in preserving life beyond this point. In particular, people sense the considerable practical and emotional burden for families in the long-term care of relatives with dementia (especially spouses), which has been confirmed in numerous studies [31]. Advanced Directives as described above, can help prevent 'heroic' yet inappropriate and unnecessary treatment should our demented selves fall gravely ill.

Emotional and spiritual care at the end of life

We have argued that fear of death on the part of the public and health professionals drives unsustainable interventions. Care that is not motivated by fear is likely then to be better, leaner and greener. Emotional care is a subtle and demanding undertaking, and something that the *Hospice Movement* has championed [32]. Much of this comes through conversations with carers who see it as their role to talk meaningfully amid the routine tasks of care such as meals, baths and transfers. There is also reference now to the *amicus mortis*, or 'friend in death', a professional or volunteer who can help 'hold' the unfolding situation with the dying person and their family and who has a similar role to that of the *doula* who supports parents through the birthing process [33]. Complementary therapies are also used in emotional care in hospices, though less so in hospitals and in the community. The more common modalities include massage, acupuncture and hypnosis. The use of massage, for instance, makes intuitive sense, especially in those deprived of touch through bereavement or hospitalisation. Fairly robust clinical evidence exists for the positive effects of massage in the treatment of pain, fatigue and anxiety in the cancer setting [34]. The use of music in end-of-life care, which can continue after linguistic abilities are lost, is a particularly intriguing field [30].

The green funeral

The cost of dying does not end with death, and many people may wish to make their funereal plans consistent with their values, like the mother quoted at the start of the chapter. The adventurous may wish to plan an entirely 'do-it-yourself' funeral. This is legal, potentially less expensive and may help bereaved people come to terms more directly with their loss. For some people the 'assembly line' atmosphere of some cremation services may be quite out of line with their values. Others will do well to contact a sympathetic funeral director who will strive to help create congruous arrangements. Cultural differences exist with respect to visiting the body after death. In Ireland, for example, it is still commonplace for the body to rest at home on the night before the funeral and for the coffin to be left open. Spending time with the body of a deceased person while all the family comes together to say a final farewell will often feel quite natural, though this has become an increasingly uncommon practice in the West.

The woodland burial

The next aspect of the Green Death is, of course, how to lay the loved one to rest. Cremation was originally seen as green but, as mentioned earlier, it consumes a lot of energy. And even with the latest technology, cremation emits pollutants into the atmosphere. Simpler coffin materials, such as cardboard or woven willow, can mitigate some of these problems. Some highly green options do exist in theory (such as composting the body over 12 weeks) and practice (for example, freeze-drying the body in liquid nitrogen) but the most practical method remains burial. Amongst options, the *woodland burial* has much to recommend it. Though relatives and friends of the deceased may have to travel some way from their immediate neighbourhood, there is an appeal to the body 'returning to earth' and (eventually) nourishing a tree planted above the remains, which are buried in a more biodegradable coffin. Woodland burial sites typically mark graves with small plaques, flush with the ground in spacious settings, designed to remain as open woodland in perpetuity. Such facilities have an amenity value unimaginable in the typical cemetery. For example, families can return to the site for picnics and other anniversary occasions. Most woodland burial facilities discourage embalming. *Memorial Woodland* in Bristol, UK, arranges only a few embalmings each year to preserve the body when, for instance, a family member is delayed in getting back to the United Kingdom for the funeral. Rather than preserving the body, the natural burial seeks to facilitate its return to the elemental cycles. As well as providing green spaces, woodland burials typically offer friends and family more time in which to carry out their ceremonies of farewell. In the United Kingdom, a municipal crematorium books services at intervals of 30 minutes, whereas centres like *Memorial Woodland* offer several hours. It may be worth reminding families that it is often possible to book longer slots at municipal crematoria for a reasonable fee. Even with a given funeral company, the cost of a funeral can vary widely, depending on what options are chosen, but the overall costs of a woodland burial are roughly equivalent to those of a conventional burial.

Policy perspectives

Policy around the care of the dying is changing. The UK's *Royal College of Nursing (RCN)* and *Royal College of General Practitioners (RCGP)* have produced a simple, short *End of Life Care Patients Charter* that puts the patient firmly at the centre of care [35]. Palliative care is now the norm rather than the exception for United Kingdom cancer patients, and because there are relatively few hospice beds, the focus has shifted to providing palliative care in the community. All this bodes well for reducing the carbon footprint of death. Unfortunately, in many low income countries palliative care services are still poorly developed and pain relief is often unavailable [36].

The role for health professionals in the move to a sustainable human society is writ large. In this chapter we have shown how our attitudes and practices around death will be central to this transition. When the medical establishment begins to see a good death as a very palpable, important and coveted goal of medical care, then a very important dialogue will have begun. This dialogue will lead to a reconfiguration of care at the end of life away from heroic intervention toward high levels of symptom control, the preservation of consciousness and the championing of a deeper engagement with the process for patients and carers. A virtuous consequence of this dialogue will be that fewer resources will be unnecessarily and inappropriately squandered on death and dying.

Action points

Personal

- Discuss our own death with family and friends.
- Record in writing personal thoughts about death.
- Create an Advanced Directive.
- Visit a crematorium and woodland burial facility.

Practice

- Obtain training in Advance Care Planning.
- Initiate Advance Care Planning discussions with patients.

- Show interest in patients who create Advance Directives.
- Advocate on behalf of patients in end-of-life care situations.
- Demonstrate clinical judgement in initiating treatments, such as PEG feeding.
- Discuss funeral and burial options with families.

Policy

- Support national campaigns such as Dying Matters in the UK.
- Advocate for palliative care services.
- Make the good death a central strand of good medical practice.

References

1. Reuters (2010) U.S. spending on plastic surgery dips to $10 billion [Internet]. http://uk.reuters.com/article/2010/04/27/us-plastic-surgery-idUKTRE63Q02P2 0100427 [accessed 10 March 2012].

2. Wienrich, S. *et al.* (2002) *After Life: Reports from the Frontline of Death.* The Natural Death Centre, London.

3. Perkins, H.S. (2000) Time To Move Advance Care Planning Beyond Advance Directives. *Chest*, **117** (5), 1228–1231.

4. *The New Yorker* (2010) Hospice medical care for dying patients [Internet]. http://www.newyorker.com/reporting/2010/08/02/100802fa_fact_gawande [accessed 1 July 2011].

5. Bishop, T.F., Federman, A.D. and Keyhani, S. (2010) Physicians' views on defensive medicine: a national survey. *Archives of Internal Medicine*, **170** (12), 1081–1083.

6. Turow, J. (1996) Television entertainment and the US health-care debate. *Lancet*, **347** (9010), 1240–1243.

7. Christakis, N.A. and Lamont, E.B. (2000) Extent and determinants of error in doctors' prognoses in terminally ill patients: prospective cohort study. *British Medical Journal*, **320** (7233), 469–472.

8. Gomes, B., Calanzani, N. and Higginson, I.J. (2011) Local preferences and place of death in regions within England 2010. Cicely Saunders International, London.

9. Kaplan, R.M. (2011) Variation between end-of-life health care costs in Los Angeles and San Diego: why are they so different? *Journal of Palliative Medicine*, **14** (2), 215–220.

10. Mitchell, Jr, J.J. (2011) The findings of the Dartmouth Atlas Project: a challenge to clinical and ethical excellence in end-of-life care. *Journal of Clinical Ethics.* **22** (3), 267–276.

11. Center to Advance Palliative Care (2011) America's Care of Serious illness: A State-by-State Report Card on Access to Palliative Care in Our Nation's Hospitals [Internet]. http://www.capc.org/reportcard/findings [accessed 8 March 2012].

12. Connor, A., Lillywhite, R. and Cooke, M.W. (2010) The carbon footprint of a renal service in the United Kingdom. *QJM*, **103** (12), 965–975.

13. Harris, M. (2008) *Grave Matters: A Journey Through the Modern Funeral Industry to a Natural Way of Burial.* Scribner Book Company.

14. Mail Online (2010) Councils to stockpile bodies to cut the cost of cremations [Internet]. http://www.dailymail.co.uk/news/article-1325033/Councils -stockpile-bodies-cut-cost-cremations.html [accessed 10 July 2011].

15. Environmental Science: Cremation – energy used, plant corn, btus [Internet]. http://en.allexperts.com/q/Environmental-Science-1471/f/Cremation-energy -used.htm [accessed 5 January 2012].

16. FBCA (The Federation Of Burial and Cremation Authorities) – Halving Mercury Emissions From Crematoria: Novel 'Burden Sharing' Approach To Continue [Internet]. http://www.fbca.org.uk/defra-oct06.asp [accessed 10 July 2011].

17. Collins, E., Kearins, K. and Tregidga, H. (2009) Exiting in a State of Grace: can death be sustainable? *International Journal of Sustainable Strategic Management*, **1** (3), 258–284.

18. Wienrich, S. (2003) *The Natural Death Handbook* (3rd Revised edn). Rider Books, London.

19. Lowry, F. (1997) Does doctors' own fear of dying hinder palliative care? *Canadian Medical Association Journal*, **157** (3), 301–302.

20. Lo, B., McLeod, G.A. and Saika, G. (1986) Patient attitudes to discussing life-sustaining treatment. *Archives of Internal Medicine*, **146** (8), 1613–1615.

21. Kellogg, F.R., Crain, M., Corwin, J. and Brickner, P.W. (1992) Life-sustaining interventions in frail elderly persons. Talking about choices. *Archives of Internal Medicine*, **152** (11), 2317–2320.

22. Boyd, K. and Murray, S.A. (2010) Recognising and managing key transitions in end of life care. *British Medical Journal*, **341**, c4863.

23. Thompson, T., Barbour, R. and Schwartz, L. (2003) Adherence to advance directives in critical care decision making: vignette study. *British Medical Journal*, **327** (7422), 1011.

24. Prommer, E.E. (2010) Using the values-based history to fine-tune advance care planning for oncology patients. *Journal of Cancer Education*, **25** (1), 66–69.

25. Cohen, R.I., Lisker, G.N., Eichorn, A., Multz, A.S. and Silver, A. (2009) The impact of do-not-resuscitate order on triage decisions to a medical intensive care unit. *Journal of Critical Care*, **24** (2), 311–315.

26. Venneman, S.S., Narnor-Harris, P., Perish, M. and Hamilton, M. (2008) 'Allow natural death' versus 'do not resuscitate': three words that can change a life. *Journal of Medical Ethics*, **34** (1) 2–6.

27. Bynum, J.PW., Andrews, A., Sharp, S., McCollough, D. and Wennberg, J.E. (2011) Fewer hospitalizations result when primary care is highly integrated into a continuing care retirement community. *Health Affairs (Millwood)*, **30** (5), 975–984.

28. Wright, A.A., Zhang, B., Ray, A. *et al.* (2008) Associations Between End-of-Life Discussions, Patient Mental Health, Medical Care Near Death, and Caregiver Bereavement Adjustment. *Journal of the American Medical Association*, **300** (14), 1665–1673.
29. Molloy, D.W., Guyatt, G.H., Russo, R. *et al.* (2000) Systematic implementation of an advance directive program in nursing homes: a randomized controlled trial. *Journal of the American Medical Association*, **283** (11), 1437–1444.
30. Aldridge, D. (1998) *Music Therapy in Palliative Care: New Voices.* Jessica Kingsley, London.
31. Murray, J., Schneider, J., Banerjee, S. and Mann, A. (1999) EUROCARE: a cross-national study of co-resident spouse carers for people with Alzheimer's disease: II – a qualitative analysis of the experience of caregiving. *International Journal of Geriatric Psychiatr,.* **14** (8), 662–667.
32. Kimberley McLaughlin, R.T. (2011) Terror and intimacy – unlocking secrets at the end of life. *Holistic Healthcare*, **8** (1) 12–17.
33. Elliott, H. (2011) Moving Beyond the Medical Model. *Holistic Healthcare*, **8** (1), 27–30.
34. Cassileth, B.R. and Vickers, A.J. (2004) Massage therapy for symptom control: outcome study at a major cancer center. *Journal of Pain Symptom Management*, **28** (3), 244–249.
35. Royal College of General Practitioners (2010) Joint RCGP and RCN End of Life Care Patient Charter [Internet]. http://www.rcgp.org.uk/end_of_life_care/patient_charter.aspx [accessed 11 June 2011].
36. Webster, R., Lacey, J. and Quine, S. (2007) Palliative care: a public health priority in developing countries. *Journal of Public Health Policy*, **28** (1), 28–39.

Chapter 11 **The Green Academy**

"Education is not the filling of a bucket, but the lighting of a fire."

WB Yeats

In this chapter

- The four quadrants of the green academy
- Integrating sustainability into the undergraduate curriculum
- Teaching methods in sustainability
- Incorporating greener working practices in healthcare

There is a pressing need to weave sustainability into healthcare education for undergraduates, postgraduates in training and the wider healthcare workforce. The current generation of students is the generation that will face the brunt of the challenges outlined in previous chapters, including those of resource depletion and climate change. Sustainability also needs to find its way onto the agenda of the major medical research institutions as we start to decipher the links between health and the environment. Meanwhile the higher education sector has its own substantive carbon footprint with, for instance, 14.6 million students enrolled in full-time higher education in the United States. Founded on principles of public service and cultural enrichment, our universities are well placed to be in the vanguard of sustainable transition.

As outlined in Chapters 1 and 3, sustainability is a paradigm, a distinct way of thinking about our place in the world. Sustainability education is, therefore, about changing perspectives as well as acquiring knowledge [1]. Currently, healthcare education equips students to function within the established system; for example, teaching them how to prescribe effectively and safely. By 'greening the gaze', sustainability education asks students to take a wider systems view, encouraging them not to take the status quo as

Sustainable Healthcare, First Edition. Knut Schroeder, Trevor Thompson, Kathleen Frith and David Pencheon.
© 2013 John Wiley & Sons, Ltd. Published 2013 by John Wiley & Sons, Ltd.

a given, but to maintain an open mind with an attitude of critical enquiry throughout their training and following career. Taking prescribing as an example, sustainability education stimulates students to question the impact of a particular medication on the patient's overall health and whether it enhances resilience, while also assessing and appreciating its wider impact on the environment. Facilitating such higher order thinking is a challenge for the current generation of Faculty who have not themselves been trained to think ecologically, but several examples of good practice are explored here.

In this chapter we start with a closer look at the university enterprise before examining the 'what' and the 'how' of sustainability in curriculum design, conferencing and research.

The university enterprise

At present, we do not normally expect educators or employers to be aware of sustainability issues. But this situation is destined to change as the century unfolds. Now is the time for higher education institutions to show vision and embed sustainability as a transparent ingredient of the overall student experience. Younger generations are variously aware that they will have to overcome the major global challenges that are predicted to emerge in the coming decades. Maybe this is why students often teem with ideas and initiatives, once given the freedom to express them. It is a pleasure to see how sustainability teaching often dissolves the usual academic hierarchies, where, due to this being a new field, students frequently teach as much as they learn. Often the job of Faculty is only to be there with enthusiasm, saying 'Yes, this matters', not filling the bucket but lighting, or at least stoking, the fire.

Teaching is of course only one aspect of university life. The UN General Assembly declared 2005–2014 the 'Decade of Education for Sustainable Development (ESD)' [2]. UNESCO has marked this decade with many ESD initiatives aimed at helping institutions achieve overall sustainability as *Green Academies*. The Green Academy comprises four quadrants: education, research, managing the estate and the 'informal curriculum' (Figure 11.1).

Education

There are two aspects to consider within the education quadrant: bringing sustainability *content* into the taught curriculum and delivering education more sustainably, irrespective of the particular content. Many universities now cover sustainability themes in their curricula and across faculties (Case study 11.1) but there is currently little sustainability teaching within health-care programmes [3]. In most countries, professional regulatory bodies

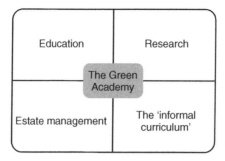

Figure 11.1 The Green Academy.

Case study 11.1 University of bristol open unit in sustainability [5]

Delivered by expert academic staff from Geographical Sciences, History, Economics, Law, Philosophy, Earth Sciences, Engineering and Education, the University of Bristol's awarding-winning Open Unit *Sustainable Development* offers students a diverse introduction to the principles, practices and problems of adopting a sustainable development (SD) approach to a wide range of human endeavours.

No 'pre' or 'co' requisites and no previous knowledge of the subject are required or assumed. Through the lecture programme, students' preconceptions of SD are challenged and they are asked to consider a range of questions from an interdisciplinary perspective, such as 'how can we address global challenges such as climate change, resource depletion, and energy security?'

---

determine educational priorities, which up to now have rarely included sustainability. In the United Kingdom, the General Medical Council (GMC) publishes guidelines for the knowledge, skills and attitudes that medical students must learn at UK medical schools in its manual 'Tomorrow's Doctors' [4]. This framework requires medical schools to 'discuss from a global perspective the determinants of health and disease' (Section 11j). At the time of writing, work is underway with the GMC to make requirements for sustainability education more explicit. Essential curricular elements are likely to include an awareness of climate science and the impact of global environmental change on health (Chapter 2) as well as an appreciation of sustainable systems, carbon literacy and the advocacy role of health professionals (Chapter 3). The *delivery* of education itself also has considerable sustainability implications. A Green Academy thinks, for instance, of how much it will require its students to travel and, aware of its carbon footprint, designs systems such as lift-shares to minimise this. This is a particular issue for clinical placements to hospitals remote to the main teaching hospital.

Research

The research quadrant also has two main aspects. Firstly, there is research on global environmental problems and their solutions. In the main, this is conducted outside the healthcare sector in departments such as geography, biology and economics but often includes health-related dimensions. There is, however, emerging research in the medical field, such as the work of the *Green Nephrology Network*, on the carbon impact of a regional nephrology service [6]. Research on sustainability in healthcare is set to expand over the coming decades and an agenda has been set out by the United Kingdom's influential *King's Fund* [7]. Secondly, there is the carbon impact of the research process, regardless of the actual nature of that research. We look at both these aspects of research in more depth later in this chapter.

Estates

The higher education sector has, like healthcare institutions, large estates to manage. Most institutions now have environmental action plans, covering areas such as procurement, waste, construction and biodiversity, ideally implemented by a dedicated management team. In the United Kingdom, universities are required under the terms of the Climate Change Act (2008) to make plans for an 80% cut in carbon emissions by 2050 [8]. To make this happen, the higher education sector needs to engage in the processes that we have already described in previous chapters relating to, for instance, transport, procurement, food and waste. In the United Kingdom, institutions can find their position on a *Green League* that ranks them according to clear criteria of green engagement [9]. These criteria include environmental policy, carbon management and ethical procurement as well as energy, water and waste performance, which are then combined into a total score. Progress will have been made when universities take their *Green League* ranking as seriously as their positions in other academic performance tables.

The informal curriculum

The informal curriculum – how students travel, eat, heat and socialise – is perhaps the area of university life that has the biggest carbon impact. It is also the hardest to define and influence. A carbon footprint study of students by *Transition Edinburgh University's Steering Group* found that only 15% of their emissions came from the institution itself, compared with 85% from the community's lifestyle [10]. However, evidence has emerged that student behaviour can be swayed by the general culture of an institution. For instance, highly visible waste recycling facilities, healthy food options, low-carbon mass transport and lecture programmes can all help to raise awareness on campus that can translate into more sustainable behaviour [11]. Some institutions have schemes, such as Bristol's *Green Impact Awards*, to harness and reward enthusiasm. Much of the initiative in the informal curriculum comes directly from student activism.

Thinking about universities in terms of these four quadrants helps us to appreciate the impact of higher education institutions inside and outside the usual academic domains of teaching and research. We turn now to the question of what should be included within a sustainable healthcare curriculum.

The sustainable healthcare curriculum

This book forms, in itself, the skeleton of a sustainable healthcare curriculum. As we have already established, more sustainable healthcare is *better* care, so curricular elements that foster quality, such as more effective prescribing or the rational ordering of investigations, may encourage sustainability without the need for any formal sustainability teaching. For example, in cardiovascular medicine it is standard practice to tackle lifestyle factors as a routine part of the management of hypertension, though guidelines continue to dwell mainly on pharmaceutical measures. However, health professionals need some specialist knowledge that is not currently included in medical curricula. This knowledge can be divided into five learning themes (Figure 11.2).

Why sustainability?

We need to provide students with an understanding of the current threats to the earth system, in particular climate change, resource depletion, wealth inequalities, the growth of human consumption/population and the loss of biodiversity (Chapter 1). Understanding these crises as systemic problems of the global economy will help students gain a nuanced understanding of how sustainability is fundamental to their solution. Students will then find it easier to appreciate the features of a healthy system in terms of responsive feedback loops, diversity and redundancy. They will also become better equipped to understand key vocabulary, such as mitigation, adaptation and the precautionary principle (Chapter 3). In the healthcare context, an understanding

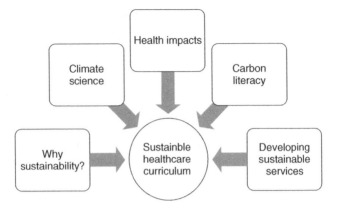

Figure 11.2 Learning outcomes within sustainable healthcare curricula.

of the centrality of preventative medicine, of building resilience and of the virtuous cycles that promote both human and planetary health will be crucial.

Climate science

A basic understanding of climate science is important for students to appreciate the size and urgency of the global problems we face. Knowledge about the mechanisms by which sustainable behaviour can mitigate the effects of global environmental change is also needed. This includes knowing about the figures on global warming in the industrial era and understanding the greenhouse effect – in particular, the role of carbon dioxide derived from fossil fuels (Chapter 2). Understanding the notion of the earth as a self-regulating system and having a sense of the history of earth's climate and how that is ascertained is core knowledge. Importantly, we need to help students appreciate the effects of global warming on ice melts, hydrological cycles and extreme weather. Learning about climate science allows students to become familiar with climate as an unpredictable, non-linear system with tipping points and the potential for rapid and potentially catastrophic change. This knowledge can often be conveyed through a single lecture combined with an online interactive tutorial.

Health impacts

It is critical that students learn to appreciate the weighty impacts of global environmental factors on human health, and climate change in particular

(Chapter 2). This includes an understanding of the public health impacts of floods, droughts, extreme weather, sea level rises and changes in the epidemiology of disease vectors. Another learning outcome for students is to appreciate the timescale over which these effects may emerge and how they will affect different regions in different ways (poorer nations in particular). This helps them comprehend the notion of food security and the global effects of mass migration from afflicted regions.

Carbon literacy

While natural resources deplete, the earth warms and legislation bites, students will benefit from becoming carbon literate and numerate with the ability to make value judgements about the merits of different sustainability interventions. For instance, the average European generates $13\,000\,kg\,CO_2e$ per annum – so an intervention that saves, say, $10\,kg\,CO_2e$, is small by comparison but considerable if repeated often. Students need a sense of what 1 kg or 1000 kg of carbon dioxide actually equates to in terms of energy used. Examples include learning to appreciate the carbon impacts of bringing a patient up for an outpatient appointment, performing an MRI scan or conducting an elective hip operation (Table 11.1). All students should be able to measure their own carbon footprints and those of services they are engaged with.

Developing sustainable services

We need to help students to understand the principles of sustainable services, including issues of travel and transport, food, procurement and

Table 11.1 The carbon footprint of some common procedures* (personal communication from Dr Adam Pollard, Research Fellow, Peninsula College of Medicine and Dentistry, UK).

Bone scan	25.1
CT scan	5.4
Fluoroscopy	16.1
Mammogram	3.2
MRI	8.3
X-ray	1.2

*all figures are kg

waste management. These can be illustrated by citing examples of best practice in settings similar to their own or, better still, by giving them scope to influence services themselves through, say, carbon audits. We should enable and encourage students to become advocates for sustainability and show leadership in driving change, using methodologies such as *Sustainable Action Planning* (which is explained later in this chapter). Since sustainable services are typically high quality services, this provides really effective lessons in commissioning and service development.

Although these five learning outcomes will have face validity for many educationalists, they naturally raise questions for practical implementation in individual institutions. These are new topics that healthcare educators are unlikely to have met in their own educational experience. But early signs are promising. Although in the United Kingdom, for instance, sustainability does not explicitly feature in the curricula of the majority of medical schools, there is a growing body of evidence and experience providing inspiration and practical assistance [12, 13].

Teaching methods

The methods for teaching the sustainability curriculum are not fundamentally different from those for teaching in any other healthcare field. In this section some current and useful practices are described.

Lectures

When it comes to conveying information about climate science or the health impacts of global environmental change, there is still a place for the traditional lecture. In this field there are many opportunities for the use of photographs and vivid graphics. The famous saw-toothed curve of atmospheric carbon dioxide from the Mauna Loa observatory is a good example (Chapter 2), as are photographs showing the retreat of glaciers, desertification and inundation. Links to pre-prepared slide shows, ripe for adaptation to local contexts, can be downloaded from the website of the *Sustainable Healthcare Education Network* [12]. Teachers who are fortunate to have access to climate scientists will do well to involve them directly in teaching. Students may be sceptical about the scientific consensus on global warming when their information is sourced from clamorous and often dichotomising newspaper headlines. Hearing about the science directly from sober authors of original research, themselves often confounded by the media, gives students confidence in the scientific foundations of sustainability – and for some this can be highly motivating. Students enjoy practical demonstrations. For instance, the systems principle that 'the whole is more than the sum of the parts' can be easily and humorously illustrated by using a *chaotic pendulum*, comprising two simple pendulums connected in series that, when given a shove, perform extraordinary and unpredictable rotational gymnastics [14].

Using film

Film is an excellent medium to convey ideas and information on climate change and sustainability, provided that teaching is structured in a way that allows subsequent group reflection and debate. A well-known and conspicuous example is Al Gore's *Inconvenient Truth*, which interweaves Gore's personal journey with hard-hitting facts on global warming. In *The Age of Stupid*, Oscar-nominated Pete Postlethwaite portrays a man living alone in the devastated world of 2055, looking back at archive footage from 2007 and asking: 'Why didn't we stop climate change when we had the chance?' *Food, Inc.*, though focused solely on the United Staes' experience, is packed with insights into the industrialisation of food production. Michael Moore's *Sicko* is a characteristically ruthless portrayal of the failings of a commercially driven health system. A large collection of freely available environmentally-themed films has been collected on the www.topdocumentaryfilms.com website. Students can watch these in class and/or submit critical reviews as part of their assessment.

World café

The *World Café* is a social technology for generating and unpacking issues in a lively and inclusive way [15]. It allows students who have gained a certain basic level of information and who will often have thought deeply on these issues to share their ideas and become more involved in the learning process. In a world café learning session, a set of learners is split into café-table sized groups and equipped with pens, paper and a unique central question or theme. Groups then unpack their themes (for instance, student lift-shares for clinical attachments) before moving on to do the same at another table, leaving behind a host to quickly brief new arrivals before the conversation proceeds. Though not a method for concrete planning, it can, when going well, release incredible creativity and enthusiasm.

Debate

Rather than offering the pretence of certainty, educators do well to actively encourage a culture of debate and enquiry. For instance, in 2007, the use of the film *Inconvenient Truth* as a teaching aid in United Kingdom schools was challenged in the High Court by a school governor and political activist, objecting to alleged inaccuracies [16]. The judge's ruling can be provided to students as fodder for debate on the media representation of climate science. Other examples of topics for debate include the motion that 'All Doctors Should be Vegetarians', which was debated by students at Leeds University Medical School with lively results. And the motion 'Medical Care Cannot be Rationed by its Carbon Costs' is also guaranteed to get students puzzling over hard questions.

Outside the classroom

Teaching about the environment often engages students more if it takes place outside, 'on location'. A simple lesson around energy consumption, for example, can easily take place in an urban setting by going to a vantage point and having students observe the sights, sounds and smells of energy being consumed – all the better with a view of a major highway. In teaching carbon literacy students can push a car a certain distance with the engine off. This typically exhausts four or five students, who can then calculate the quantity of petrol (gas) required to move the same distance: a nice illustration of the amount of energy embedded in hydrocarbons. It can also be enlightening to (safely) combust a pint (568 ml) of petrol; the impressive conflagration emits almost exactly 1 kg of carbon dioxide. This output can be compared to that of common products. For instance, a typical cheeseburger is responsible for the emission of 2.5 kg of carbon dioxide. Many pharmaceutical companies will allow students to visit their manufacturing sites, where it is intrinsically interesting to see how medicines are made. Visiting such sites can also help students understand how seriously some companies consider ways to save energy.

The business pitch (or 'Dragon's Den')

Based on the format of the BBC television programme *Dragon's Den*, in which entrepreneurs pitch business ideas to wealthy and fault-finding financiers, students can present ideas for new or improved clinical services to an audience of peers or invited experts. The challenge for students in such a lesson is to show how they have weaved sustainability thinking into their proposals. This model has been used by teachers at Leicester University Medical School and shown to get students thinking about the complexities of commissioning.

Direct action projects

An inspirational and effective way to deliver learning around sustainability management and advocacy is to have students run their own project on or off campus. At Leeds University, for instance, medical students have gone into sixth form colleges to teach about the potential health consequences of climate change. At Bristol University, students jumped through many bureaucratic hoops to run a farmer's market right outside the university's senate building. Their market included information stalls and through their trailblazing the university now hosts a market every fortnight. In a highly creative awareness raising campaign, two students cycled through a one hour lecture and demonstrated that their efforts created only enough energy to light and heat the lecture theatre for 20 minutes. Direct action projects face students with the challenges of indifference and denial as well as giving them a real sense of achievement.

Organisations supporting sustainability education

In designing education for sustainability there are many organisations to draw on for inspiration, information, advice and teaching resources. In the United Kingdom, for example, there is the *Sustainable Healthcare Education Network (SHE)*, hosted by the *Centre for Sustainable Healthcare*. This network brings together medical clinicians, academics and students to develop, pilot and share teaching materials specifically designed to bring a sustainability 'perspective' to the medical curriculum and to the UK General Medical Councils' 'Tomorrow's Doctors' learning outcomes. A link to educational materials from the SHE is included at the end of this chapter. In the United States, the *Centre for Health and the Global Environment* at Harvard University aims to present the best and most current science about the environment and human health in non-technical language that is easy to understand, not only for students and physicians but also for scientists, policymakers and the general public [17]. This field has also seen the recent emergence of journals devoted to the topic, such as The *Journal of Sustainability Education* and the *International Journal of Sustainability in Higher Education*. These journals provide a forum for educators, practitioners and researchers to share and critique ideas with many articles specifically relating to health themes.

Sustainability in medical research

As with education there are two distinct aspects to consider: firstly, research on the greening of the healthcare enterprise and, secondly, the need to make the actual doing of medical research more sustainable, regardless of the topic. We cover both aspects in this section. Sustainability has not traditionally been the concern of medical researchers, though this will change as major grant awarding bodies begin to appreciate the health impacts of global environmental change. In 2012 the UK's King's Fund published a report exploring the research agenda for sustainable healthcare, commissioned by the UK government, and its proposals are wide-ranging [7]. It advocates more research into preventative medicine, co-benefits (virtuous cycles), the environmental costs of specific interventions, leaner medicines management and self-care for chronic conditions. It also advocates research into individual and organisational behaviour, including barriers to change, sustainable commissioning and ways of better engaging professionals and public in this agenda.

We also need to think about the carbon impact of the medical research process, which has itself become a subject of investigation. For example, a carbon audit of two clinical trials quantified the carbon emissions produced over one year and concluded that faster patient recruitment led to greatly increased carbon efficiency in terms of emissions per randomised patient. The impacts from travel related to various aspects of the trial were shown to be particularly high because of the trial team commuting to work (21 tonnes of carbon dioxide per trial), fuel use within trial centres (18 tonnes), trial-related travel (15 tonnes) and travel from study participants (13 tonnes) [18].

These data highlight the need for the research community to take sustainability considerations into account when designing and conducting research, be it basic research, drug trials or research into services. The UK National Institute for Health Research has produced a framework which identifies areas where better research design can minimise waste without negatively impacting on the reliability and validity of studies [19]. Its report identifies six key areas (Figure 11.3).

Setting the research question should make full use of existing evidence and involve clinicians as well as healthcare users. Studies are more effective if they make best use of resources (for instance, relating to time and travel), try to answer more than one question within one study (for example, through a factorial trial design) and involve research methodologists from an early stage. Collaborating with research networks and other researchers, and working directly with people involved in recruiting participants (such as clinicians, patients and administrative staff), can help optimise procedures. Avoiding unnecessary data collection is paramount and, where possible, outcomes should be measured remotely by using technologies such as the telephone or the Internet. Inefficient monitoring procedures, such as unnecessary site visits, should be avoided. Good practice in reporting research includes presenting study results in the context of updated systematic reviews of previous relevant research. This helps to ensure that research publications and reports contain information that is of direct relevance to readers. As with clinical care, research done more efficiently is intrinsically greener.

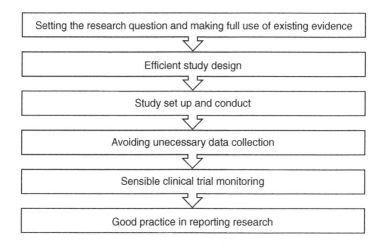

Figure 11.3   Six key areas for making research more sustainable [19].

To facilitate this process, sustainability needs to be formally cited at the heart of research governance, so that researchers are held to account with measures such as 'Potential health gain per tonne of carbon expended' or 'Patients recruited per tonne of CO_2e' [20]. *Practice Greenhealth* has developed a web-based *Energy Impact Calculator* that fits this description [21]. The research community (including funders, commissioners and distributors of research) is in a good position to set an example to the wider healthcare community. Examples of major international journals that take sustainability issues seriously are, among others, the *American Journal of Preventive Medicine*, the *British Medical Journal* and the *Lancet*.

The green conference

Attending medical conferences can be inspirational. It can also be a dispiriting experience with delegates spending the majority of their time sitting passively through series of presentations. In keeping with what we know of healthy systems, conferences can provide various types of opportunities for delegates to connect with each other and to the ideas that are important to them. Mostly it is the people we meet and conversations we join that make a particular conference memorable, along with perhaps an impressive keynote speech.

However, some of the things that make taking part in conferences so useful are routinely replicable through web-based technologies, which are well adapted to help people network and learn from each other beyond geographical limitations. An example is the collection of cutting-edge lectures at www.ted.com, which includes many on medical themes. We are also just starting to appreciate the potential of the *webinar*, a live online seminar format that can include a slideshow, text chat, whiteboard annotation and a recording for posterity. As we tighten our carbon belts, such types of conference will inevitably become more commonplace.

Perhaps we ought to set limits to how much health professionals, particularly doctors, travel for medical conferences – another good topic for a student debate. For instance, health professionals may make conference trips not because they really wish to confer but because they need to disseminate their research. Where this is the case, research presentations are often ideally suited to teleconferencing from the home institution. International conferences, where people fly in for brief visits, are highly carbon intensive. For instance, the total carbon dioxide emissions for flying the 15 000 delegates to and from the American Thoracic Society international conference in May 2006 was an estimated 10 779 tons [22]. It would take an average American adult 200 years to generate an equivalent amount in their personal life [23].

Where the face-to-face encounter is the most desirable option, much can be done to make conferences more sustainable. An article by the UK's National Health Executive published in 2011 provides some succinct guidance for teaching and training events, as summarised in Figure 11.4 [24].

Here are some ideas around how these strategies can work in practice.

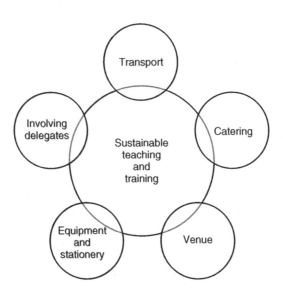

Figure 11.4 Areas to consider for making training models more sustainable (adapted from National Health Executive 2011) [24].

Transport

Walk the talk by choosing locations that are easily accessible by public transport or through active travel, saving travel time and costs. To make sure that participants book the most effective routes and means of travel, provide comprehensive travel information in your pre-course information sheet. Consider incentivising sustainable travel with fee discounts to get more people signed up to sustainable travel and make things as easy as possible for cyclists by signposting them to bike storage and shower facilities. To help the planning of future events, collect information from participants about the way they travelled.

Venue

When choosing a training venue, give preference to locations with lots of fresh air and natural light. A venue which uses renewable sources to provide the energy for electricity, heating and cooling is itself a lesson in sustainability. Whenever possible, use venues within or close to natural environments, such as parks or gardens.

Catering

At the event, offer fresh, unprocessed and locally produced food. Supply jugs with tap water and avoid bottled water. Where using local supplies, display details of producers to stimulate interest and conversation. Make your catering policy explicit in your paperwork and in announcements on the day. Investigate the use of reusable service dishes and cutlery. Because eating together is such an important social aspect of a meeting or conference, attention to the catering can have a surprisingly important influence on the feel of the whole event. And, of course, do not waste food.

Equipment

Avoid printed material and ideally provide information, handouts and other course materials electronically through email or a website. If you need to print material, prevent duplication and print on both sides of recycled paper, using the 'fast' print setting. Use writing material made of recycled material where possible and make sure you recycle any left-over paper or flip charts.

Involving delegates

Use opportunities to raise sustainability awareness among delegates, for example by pointing out any reductions in waste that you have achieved and the costs (and, better, cost savings) that are involved. Obtain feedback and ask for suggestions of how to make an event even more sustainable the next time. Consider offering rebates or prizes for the best ideas and for those who travelled in the most sustainable way.

The most effective arena for educational interventions to improve sustainability may not lie in formal courses or fancy conferences. It is often work done directly with the healthcare workforce 'on the ground'. People making up the workforce are the ones who use the resources, who can see where the potential for better stewardship lies and who can put leaner ideas directly into action.

Engaging the workforce

We will know that we are making progress when sustainability figures as highly in people's thinking as considerations of infection control or racial discrimination do now. This requires leadership and vision, not least at the top of organisations [25]. Training opportunities for senior managers are now becoming available, for instance at the *Cambridge Programme for Sustainability Leadership* [26]. Organisations can demonstrate their commitment by including sustainability and carbon governance as responsibilities on job descriptions at all levels, including those of Chief Executives and Directors [27]. A good start is to make sustainability a routine part of staff induction. Other practical measures include, for instance, adding sustainability statements onto travel expense forms, with questions such as 'Could this journey have been avoided by using teleconferencing or videoconferencing?'. There is a good case for reversely incentivising the ownership of high emission vehicles by paying a flat rate of compensation for road travel.

Using a classic resource efficiency method, the team at the Royal Cornwall Hospital Renal Unit (UK) identified carbon reduction opportunities, prioritised them and moved into action [28]. By the end of the first year it had achieved clear improvements in the patient experience with nearly 50% less waiting, fewer aborted journeys and more self-care, an improved workplace for staff with more time to look after patients (and better attendance), a reduction in healthcare acquired infections and 'cost avoidances' running at £1200 (US$ 1858) per employee per year. Aborted ambulance journeys were reduced to zero, saving £1500 (US$ 2323) per month. After two years, total yearly cost avoidance was running at £57 500 (US$ 89 033), saving over 52 tonnes of carbon in the process.

Case study 11.2 gives an example of what can be achieved through concerted strategic action in a larger publicly funded healthcare organisation [29].

Sustainable action planning

Sustainable Action Planning (SAP), designed by the *Centre for Sustainable Healthcare*, is a social technology for developing sustainability within

Case study 11.2 Sustainability benefits of wider organisational change [29]

Partly through involving its staff, the Derby Hospitals Foundation Trust (UK) it lowered the hospitals' energy consumption and carbon emissions by nearly 4%, saving over £5 million (US$ 7.7 million) in the process over a period of five years. Instrumental in this achievement was its *Earthbeat* magazine supplement 'keeping you informed on green issues', which kept staff informed about developments with the hospital on recycling, cycle to work schemes and energy saving. By appointing volunteer members of staff as 'environmental champions', the hospital managed to feed back important messages at ward and departmental level, which helped to create an interactive network across the service. This contributed to the creation an atmosphere that fostered sharing of ideas and raising awareness of sustainability issues. The Trust also raises awareness about waste, energy costs and water saving through over 100 trained Environmental Champions – enthusiastic people who help organising events and putting up posters and reminding people 'to turn off the lights'.

healthcare organisations of any size [30]. SAP aims, among other things, to increase a team's knowledge and awareness of environmental issues and support them in creating and following a green action plan. SAP empowers healthcare teams to explore together opportunities for improving their service and to come up with their own solutions, thereby establishing a new sustainability culture.

So how does SAP work? First of all, organisations need to invest time in the initiative [30]. External facilitators lead to better outcomes and prove cost effective. The intervention centres on two workshops. The first raises awareness of the global issues and helps the participants to identify possibilities and priorities for improving sustainability. In the second workshop the team uses a variety of trusted change management approaches to make concrete plans for action on its chosen priorities. Finally, SAP provides clear guidance on how to monitor and sustain the initiative.

The role of professional organisations

While action within individual organisations is critical, so, too, is leadership from national and international organisations. At the top of the tree are those that set the standards for professional practice and for what should be taught in medical and nursing colleges. A consultation process is already underway to create recommendations for the UK's General Medical Council to refer explicitly to sustainability in its guidance to doctors and medical schools. With sustainability firmly established in *Tomorrow's Doctors*, medical schools can start diverting creative and fiscal resources to the challenge. Imagine also if doctors had sustainability added to the list of criteria through which they navigate their annual appraisals. Along with headings such as 'working with others', 'maintaining clinical knowledge' and 'probity', doctors would gather evidence for their contributions to the sustainability of their practice.

Of great importance is the position taken by professional umbrella organisations such as the *British Medical Association (BMA)* and the *American Medical Association (AMA)*, or speciality associations such as the UK Royal Colleges. The UK's *Royal College of General Practitioners (RCGP)*, for instance, has a ratified sustainability policy and appointed a Sustainability Lead. Sustainability now features in the professional entry examination for general practitioners (nMRCGP) and was the core theme of the RCGP's 2010 conference. The *British Medical Journal (BMJ)* has shown commitment to the issue over many years, as has the *Lancet* [31].

Various other organisations also focus specifically on increasing sustainability in healthcare. *Health Care Without Harm*, for example, is an international coalition of hospitals and healthcare systems, medical professionals, community groups, health-affected constituencies, labour unions, environmental and environmental health organisations and religious groups. It works to implement ecologically sound and healthy alternatives to healthcare practices that pollute the environment and contribute to disease. The *NHS Sustainable Development Unit (SDU)* in England aims to help the NHS fulfil its potential as a leading sustainable and low-carbon healthcare service by developing organisations, people, tools, policy and research which will enable the NHS to promote sustainable development and mitigate climate change. The *Centre for Sustainable Healthcare* (formerly known as the *Campaign for Greener Healthcare*) is inspiring people to realise the vital importance of the overlap between their wellbeing and environmental sustainability, particularly in the field of healthcare. Various other sustainability networks exist, some of which are listed at the end of this chapter.

Turning night into day

Bringing sustainability into focus when working with all generations of healthcare staff has the potential to transform the health sector for the benefit of all. Many people working in healthcare – from anaesthetists to managers, from cleaners to kitchen staff – are already aware of the links between a healthy environment and health for people. Around the world we can see exceptional examples of ways in which healthcare can become

Box 11.1   Further information sources

- Center for Health and the Global Environment, http://chge.med.harvard.edu
- Centre for Sustainable Healthcare, http://sustainablehealthcare.org.uk. For resources from the Sustainable Healthcare Education Network see: http://sustainablehealthcare.org.uk/sustainable-healthcare-medical-schools
- Climate and Health Council, www.climateandhealth.org
- NHS Sustainable Development Unit, www.sdu.nhs.uk
- 10:10 Campaign, www.1010global.org
- Doctors for the environment, http://dea.org.au
- Schumacher College, www.schumachercollege.org.uk
- Second Nature, www.secondnature.org/
- The New Economics Foundation, www.neweconomics.org
- The Journal of Sustainability Education, www.jsedimensions.org/ojs/index.php/jse
- The Environmental Association for Universities and Colleges, www.eauc.org.uk/education_for_sustainable_development

more sustainable. What is, yet, still missing is the *critical mass*, that is, a large enough number of people within health systems who can turn such aspirations into service reality. What we can see is a night sky of stars, with each star representing outstanding initiative, innovation and performance. Unfortunately, this sky is still dark. We still have a long way to go on this journey before we can make such outstanding practice the norm in a consistent and systematic way across health services around the world, turning this dark night sky into daylight. How we can create the daylight that we need for more sustainable healthcare is part of the final chapter.

Sustainability networks

Further information, resources and useful networks are available through various organisations (Box 11.1).

References

1. Goodman, B. (2011) The need for a 'sustainability curriculum' in nurse education. *Nurse Education Today*, **31** (8), 733–737.

2. The Higher Education Academy (2011) 2011: Green Academy: Curricula for tomorrow [Internet]. http://www.heacademy.ac.uk/projects/detail/esd/esd _green_academy [accessed 15 April 2012].
3. Kirk, M. (2002) The impact of globalization and environmental change on health: challenges for nurse education. *Nurse Education Today*, **22** (1), 60–71, 72–75.
4. General Medical Council (2009) Tomorrow's Doctors [Internet]. http:// www.gmc-uk.org/education/undergraduate/tomorrows_doctors.asp [accessed 15 April 2012].
5. Hoare, A., Cornell, S., Bertram, C. *et al.* (2008) Teaching against the grain: multi-disciplinary teamwork effectively delivers a successful undergraduate unit in sustainable development. *Environmental Education Research*, **14** (4), 469–481.
6. Connor, A., Lillywhite, R. and Cooke, M.W. (2010) The carbon footprint of a renal service in the United Kingdom. *QJM*, **103** (12), 965–975.
7. Appleby, J. and Naylor, C. (2012) Environmentally Sustainable health and social care: Scoping Review. King's Fund, London.
8. Climate Change Act 2008. http://www.legislation.gov.uk/ukpga/2008/27/part/1 [accessed 19 April 2012].
9. People & Planet – People & Planet Green League [Internet]. http://people andplanet.org/greenleague [accessed 19 April 2012].
10. Transition Edinburgh University (2009) Footprints and Handprints: the Edinburgh University community's climate impact and how we can begin reducing it [Internet]. http://www.transitionedinburghuni.org.uk/files/Keynote summary.pdf [accessed 19 April 2012].
11. SAS Institute – Manchester Business School succeeds with SAS [Internet]. http://www.sas.com/success/manchester-business-school.html [accessed 19 April 2012].
12. Centre for Sustainable Healthcare – Sustainable Healthcare Education [Internet]. http://sustainablehealthcare.org.uk/sustainable-healthcare-education [accessed 25 September 2011].
13. EAUC: The Environmental Association for Universities and Colleges (Home) [Internet]. Available from: http://www.eauc.org.uk/home [accessed 19 April 2012].
14. YouTube – Chaotic 1,2 pendulum [Internet]. http://www.youtube.com/watch? v=2JzMJNMYbRw [accessed 19 April 2012].
15. Welcome to the World Café! (Home) [Internet]. http://www.theworldcafe.com/ [accessed 19 April 2012].
16. The Guardian (2007) Gore's climate film has scientific errors – judge | Environment | [Internet]. http://www.guardian.co.uk/environment/2007/oct/11/clima techange [accessed 19 April 2012].
17. The Center for Health and the Global Environment (Harvard Medical School) (Home) [Internet]. http://chge.med.harvard.edu/ [accessed 19 April 2012].
18. Lyle, K., Dent, L., Bailey, S., Kerridge, L., Roberts, I. and Milne, R. (2009) Carbon cost of pragmatic randomised controlled trials: retrospective analysis of sample of trials. *British Medical Journal*, **339**, b4187.

19. NIHR (2010) Carbon Reduction Guidelines [Internet]. http://www.nihr.ac.uk/ publications/Pages/carbon_reduction_guidelines.aspx [accessed 24 September 2011].

20. Pencheon, D.C. (2011) Managing the environmental impact of research. *Trials*, **12**, 80.

21. EIC Healthcare Energy Impact Calculator (Home) [Internet]. http://www .eichealth.org/ [accessed 1 August 2011].

22. Callister, M.E.J. and Griffiths, M.J.D. (2007) The carbon footprint of the American Thoracic Society meeting. *American Journal of Respiratory and Critical Care Medicine*, **175** (4), 417.

23. Berners-Lee, M. (2010) *How Bad Are Bananas?: The carbon footprint of everything*. Profile Books, London.

24. National Health Executive (2011) Low-carb NHS: Training and CPD for a sustainable health system [Internet]. http://content.yudu.com/A1shnw/NHEmayjune 2011/resources/index.htm?referrerUrl=http%3A%2F%2Fwww.nationalhealth executive.com%2Farchive.htm [accessed 20 September 2011].

25. NHS Sustainable Development Unit – Building Leadership Skills for Sustainable Development and a Low Carbon NHS [Internet]. http://www.sdu .nhs.uk/documents/publications/1232893824_hwdx_4_leadership_skills_for _sustainable_development_(.pdf [accessed 25 September 2011].

26. Cambridge Programme for Sustainability Leadership – Corporate Social Responsibility Training [Internet]. http://www.cpsl.cam.ac.uk/ [accessed 14 December 2011].

27. NHS. Sustainable Development Unit (2009) Saving Carbon, Improving Health: Carbon Reduction Strategy for England. Cambridge: NHS Sustainable Development Unit, Cambridge.

28. The Centre for Sustainable Healthcare (2011) Renal Unit, Royal Cornwall Hospital [Internet]. http://sap.greenerhealthcare.org/royal-cornwall-hospital -renal-unit [accessed 26 July 2011].

29. Derby Hospitals Foundation Trust [Internet]. http://www.derbyhospitals.nhs.uk/ search/?q=carbon [accessed 25 September 2012].

30. The Centre for Sustainable Healthcare – What is Sustainable Action Planning (SAP)? [Internet]. http://sap.greenerhealthcare.org/ [accessed 14 December 2011].

31. Patrick, K. (2011) Sustainable Healthcare: Getting more from less. *British Medical Journal*, **342**, d2425.

Chapter 12 **The journey towards sustainable healthcare**

In this chapter

- Is the health sector ready to act?
- Approaching sustainable development in healthcare
- Making change happen

Living and working more sustainably not only allows us to pass a liveable planet on to future generations, but also to live better in the here and now, with better health, more social equality, improved financial stability and a renewed sense of physical security. We have explored these issues throughout the book. Examples include more active travel, such as walking and cycling to move our bodies instead of letting fossil fuels do it for us, or using better ways of growing better food for better diets. Both active travel and better food help support a sustainable future while improving health today. We have learnt about the rationale and vision for sustainable development in the earlier parts of the book. In this chapter, we highlight some important steps that we need to take if we want to help make effective and global sustainable development a reality. We then describe a route for this journey, starting from where we are now.

Sustainability is not just about carbon reduction – although this is a pressing priority right now. To achieve global transition, we need a whole systems approach that helps us move towards a more sustainable and fairer world where individuals live in communities that are independent, interdependent and cohesive (Chapter 3) [1]. Perhaps the key step will be a move from a high intensity medical industry that focuses on treating diseases to one that concentrates more on preventing illness and supporting people to live well and proactively with multiple and long-standing conditions [2].

Sustainable Healthcare, First Edition. Knut Schroeder, Trevor Thompson, Kathleen Frith and David Pencheon.
© 2013 John Wiley & Sons, Ltd. Published 2013 by John Wiley & Sons, Ltd.

The journey toward sustainable healthcare has already begun around the world, but still more people and organisations need to engage with its multiple benefits to make a real difference [3, 4].

The health professions are ready to act

Healthcare providers have privileged access to their staff, patients, suppliers and their many partner organisations. The voices calling for the health sector to wake up to the challenges presented throughout this book are becoming louder. For example, the *International Council of Nurses (ICN)*, the *World Federation of Public Health Associations* and the *Centers for Disease Control and Prevention* have been urging health professionals to act against climate change and engage in more sustainable practices [5–7]. Yet despite unequivocal climate science and the clear consequences of global environmental change on health, health professionals are still not well represented at international climate change talks [8]. Paradoxically, health professionals are not the most active proponents of sustainability and seem as capable of denial as the rest of society. One possible reason for this inaction is the idea of *moral offset*. Researchers in the field of moral psychology report that subjects are 'least likely to scrutinize the moral implications of their behaviours (. . .) right after their moral self has experienced a boost from a good deed' [9]. As people working in the health sector spend their time improving people's health, they may feel they do not need to add 'improving planetary health' to their list of responsibilities.

But there is reason to be optimistic: several medical organisations now exist that specifically devote themselves to promoting sustainability in healthcare, including *Healthcare Without Harm*, the UK's *NHS Sustainable Development Unit* and the *Climate and Health Council* [10, 11]. Crucially, this agenda extends its scope beyond health structures (mainly hospitals) to *health systems*. The aims are clear: to foster greater ecological sustainability without compromising patient care or causing harm to public health and the environment [12]. Current areas of work include ten goals (Figure 12.1), all of which are covered in preceding chapters [10].

The mood within health services towards sustainability issues may be changing. For example, the NHS in England conducted a consultation in 2008 on carbon reduction. Findings were unexpectedly positive: people working in NHS organisations seemed willing and ready to engage. When asked '*Do you think the NHS should be a leading public sector sustainable and low-carbon organisation?*', 3078 out of 3279 people (94%) responding to the poll voted 'yes'. And in a 2012 national public survey on sustainability, 92% of people said they wanted the NHS to be more sustainable, with 33% stating that this should be done even if it would cost the health service

Leadership	• Prioritise environmental health
Chemicals	• Substitute harmful chemicals with safer alternatives
Waste	• Reduce, treat and safely dispose of healthcare waste
Energy	• Implement energy efficiency and clean, renewable energy generation
Water	• Reduce hospital water consuption and supply potable water
Transport	• Improve transport strategies for patients and staff
Food	• Purchase and serve sustainably grown, healthy food
Pharmaceuticals	• Safely manage and dispose of pharmaceuticals
Buildings	• Support green and healthy hospital design and construction
Purchasing	• Buy safer and more sustainable products and materials

Figure 12.1   The ten goals of the Global Environmental Health Agenda for Hospitals [10].

money [13]. This is in line with findings from research with members of the public showing that people are concerned about climate change and willing to address the perceived threats – although sustainability as a priority rates lower than other pressing issues such as jobs, security or education (Chapter 3) [14].

Strategies for sustainable development

So what, then, is the best way forward? The *Forum for the Future* and the *NHS Sustainable Development Unit* have explored ways of moving towards more sustainable healthcare provision in their document, *Fit for the Future – Scenarios for low-carbon healthcare 2030* (Chapter 4) [15]. The key recommendations from this document include the following five steps:

1. Supporting patient empowerment and appropriate participatory self-care.
2. Greater use of information technology.
3. Finding the low-carbon/high quality of life sweet spot.
4. Health promotion rather than treating illness.
5. Healthcare taking a leadership role in change.

The next sections summarise and revise some of the key issues in this area, which we have already explored in the preceding chapters.

Championing self-care

Health services have a great opportunity to help people and communities become more resilient by educating them about health, healthy living and supported self-care [16–18]. Appropriate self-care not only empowers patients but also saves costs and supports sustainable development through reducing unnecessary, expensive, inconvenient and potentially unsafe interventions. This is a key element of the *resilience* referred to in Chapter 3 – resilience not only of individuals, families and the wider community but also of health systems. In its report on *Helping People Help Themselves*, the UK *Health Foundation* identified a number of components that work well to support self-management; these range from passive information provision to initiatives that support behaviour change more actively (Box 12.1) [19].

As discussed in Chapter 5, contraception is another important area where giving people more choices can make a useful contribution towards sustainable development. By making contraceptive services more widely available and informing people about contraceptive options, health systems play an important role in reducing the number of unwanted pregnancies and, thereby, contribute to addressing the issue of over-population.

Better use of ICT

Using information and communication technology (ICT) for patient care, such as the telephone, email and telemedicine (making use of remote

---

Box 12.1 Ways to support self-management [19]

1. Involve people in making decisions.
2. Help people with problem solving.
3. Develop care plans and create a partnership between service users and professionals.
4. Promote healthy lifestyles and educate people about their conditions, including how to self-manage.
5. Motivate people to self-manage.
6. Help people to monitor their symptoms and know when to take appropriate action.
7. Help people to manage the social, emotional and physical impacts of their conditions.
8. Provide opportunities for sharing and learning from other service users.
9. Follow up proactively.

consultations via a video link or monitoring patients at a distance), reduce travel-related carbon emissions and can also improve access to services for those who find it difficult to travel. ICT can be convenient to use for both patients and health professionals, particularly where people can access healthcare from their home or workplace (without having to take time off or organise childcare) and where health professionals can assess, monitor and treat conditions effectively. For instance, a regional renal unit in England used to invite patients to attend in person for their routine reviews. Now blood samples and basic observations are taken in the community and follow-up is conducted by telephone as appropriate [20]. Although traditional advanced technologies are widely available, they have not yet been widely implemented. Increasing the use of the telephone and other telemedicinal devices for providing clinical care is likely to need a change of culture – perhaps more so from professionals than from the public. We are understandably reluctant to give up the rewards of the face-to-face encounter.

Promoting health promotion

Shifting the focus from treating disease to addressing the causes (and causes of causes) of health problems is one of the hallmarks of sustainable health-care (Chapter 5) [2]. Traditionally, funding for public health and preventive medicine has been neglected, with acute services receiving a dispropor-tionately higher fraction of resources. In England, for example, prevention expenditure in 2006/2007 was estimated at £3.7 billion (US$ 5.8 billion), which translated into only 4.0% of the total health budget – though this was higher than the OECD average of 2.8% [21]. Increasing tax on cigarettes and alcohol, mass media campaigns and brief interventions delivered by primary care clinicians have been shown to perform particularly well. Other interventions, such as getting people to exercise more, preventing road traffic collisions, improving housing and creating better access to food and water also have significant health benefits that reduce the need for costly acute medical care [22–24].

Leading by example

The healthcare community can exert influence, not only on its own work-force but also on partner organisations and on the people it serves. Because responding to global environmental challenges has now clearly been recog-nised as an essential public health function, the need for health professionals to lead by example has become stronger than ever. The *American Journal of Public Health* and other journals have devoted theme issues to the topic, while the *British Medical Journal* deals with the topic of climate change on a continuing basis [25–27].

Preparing our systems

Because of the crises that we have outlined in Chapters 1 and 2, health systems around the world need to be able to adapt effectively when they are affected by environmental events or scarce resources. In other words, we need to become resilient – a concept that was explored in Chapter 3. Case study 12.1 gives examples of lessons learnt from hurricane 'Katrina' [28].

During environmental emergencies, public health bodies and departments will usually be in charge of evaluating and communicating health risks and recommending appropriate actions [29, 30]. But rather than waiting for advice in times of crisis, healthcare organisations need to prepare for events such as heat waves, floods, fires, windstorms and droughts, as well as the effects of resource depletion, including water scarcity and peak oil. We also need to plan how to meet the health needs of migrant populations fleeing areas of plummeting food security. The *United Nations International Strategy for Disaster Reduction* provides useful guidance on how we can set

---

Case study 12.1   Lessons learnt from hurricane 'Katrina' [28]

Hurricane Katrina devastated hundreds of thousands of families in Louisiana and Mississippi, USA, in 2005, destroying houses and separating family members without adequate means of communication. Many people suffered post-traumatic stress reactions – vulnerable people in particular. Mental health services at the time were unable to cope with the surge in demand and could not meet people's immediate needs. An illuminating article by Madrid and Grant describes the mental health needs of people affected by this environmental disaster and the steps that were taken to develop sustainable mental health programs that could meet this unprecedented level of need over time [28]. A key element of providing effective disaster relief is to meet the needs not only of vulnerable people but also those of all those individuals who are responsible for their care, such as parents, teachers, guardians and health professionals. Giving attention to the long-term mental and physical health needs of disaster victims, and vulnerable people in particular, is a crucial aspect of preparing for natural and other disasters.

up our health services for managing disasters as an integral part of an overall organisational strategy [31].

Health services can play a particular role in preventing diseases and health problems that are exacerbated by climate change, which requires that we have sufficient financial and human resources. Effective disease prevention includes adequate staff training and continuing surveillance as well as being part of wider prevention and control programmes that are relevant to our particular location and situation [32].

Making sustainable healthcare happen

Although increasing numbers of healthcare professionals engage in sustainability, many are still unaware of the numerous benefits and do not yet contribute to the necessary debates and actions. The reasons for us not to fully engage in sustainability include that we may think we are too busy to get involved, perhaps feel guilty about our own current 'wasteful' practices and do not want to admit them, or are possibly 'addicted' to our current status quo of a high-carbon lifestyle, so that we feel threatened by the need for letting go of unsustainable habits. Or, as we have argued before, we may simply hold the view that because we are already doing socially worthy things, we are absolved from too much responsibility when it comes to getting involved in broader societal and civic actions that promote global health and equity (what we referred to as *moral offset*) [9, 33]. But we hope to have shown throughout this book that the reasons for thinking and acting more sustainably are really compelling. Hopefully, we have also dispelled some of the myths around sustainable development and made clear that sustainability is very much about gaining benefits rather than depriving us of the things we have come to enjoy. Although we still need a seismic shift in attitudes and behaviour to make a real difference, the signs are there that positive, effective and lasting change might after all be possible. This possibility, together with the many 'win–wins' (or co-benefits) on the way to achieving sustainability is what makes engaging in sustainable development currently so exciting.

The sustainability journey has analogies with other societal issues such as cholera, tobacco and HIV, which also create massive public challenges to which we need to respond with a change of behaviours, attitudes, governance standards and expectations on a larger scale. However, sustainability is different in that it is a part of *every* activity on the planet – and time is not on our side. We evoke here the *precautionary principle*, in which the burden of proof falls on those enacting potential harms. As the *Rio Declaration* notes: 'In order to protect the environment, the precautionary approach shall be widely applied by States according to their capabilities. Where there are threats of serious or irreversible damage, lack of full scientific certainty shall not be used as a reason for postponing cost-effective measures to prevent environmental degradation' [34].

Creating route maps towards sustainable health

The UK *NHS Sustainable Development Unit* launched in 2011 a *Route Map for Sustainable Health*, which outlines a strategy for the NHS in England to play a leading role in the journey to a lower carbon and more sustainable society [35]. This route map provides a framework for the health sector to encourage discussion and debate, as well as collaboration and coordinated action, and has been developed in collaboration with over 70 organisations, ranging from the *Association of Chartered Accountants* to the *World Health Organization*. The route map lays out a process of transition that features various goals and shifts [35]:

- From curative to preventative healthcare.
- From a specific sickness service to a culture of wellbeing.
- From professionals 'on top' to 'on tap'.
- From functional buildings to healing environments.
- From sustainable structures to sustainable systems.
- From valuing only individuals now to valuing everyone and the future in the interest of all.

  (adapted from UK Sustainable Development Unit (SDU) Route Map) [35]

It is not, however, a step-by-step guide but rather lays out three broad phases – 'getting started', 'transition' and 'transformation' – by 2050 (Figure 12.2).

From 'getting started' to 'transition' and 'transformation'

The first step is about engaging people. We all need to appreciate the scientific evidence showing that the earth system is under stress and understand how these pressures can be mitigated [35]. Such first steps in awareness are important, not because they have a large impact in themselves, but as entry points that give us the confidence that further investment of time and energy might be worthwhile. 'Killer facts', like the many offered in Chapters 1 and 2, can often hit home at this stage. This resonates with the addictions field, where the first necessary shift is from a pre-contemplative to a contemplative perspective (Chapter 3). In the *transition phase*, we

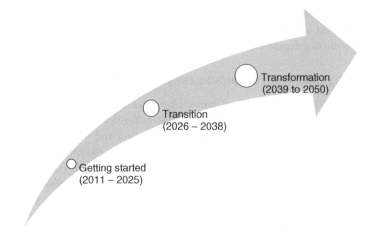

Figure 12.2   NHS Milestones towards sustainable health. (Data from [35].)

struggle and juggle with integrating sustainability into our firmly established traditional ways of doing things. The term *transition* is well chosen; it features prominently in sustainability literature and practice, including the *Transition Town* movement [36]. Edinburgh has declared itself the UK's first 'Transition University' [37]. These are all efforts to get beyond idealism and start 'from where we are' in the transition to 'what we might be'. At the time of *transformation*, sustainability will have become fully integrated into our routines, culturally embedded in our work and personal lives, and regulating itself with little need for external control. Although some of these phases unfold into the future, preparing for and achieving them requires immediate action.

Evaluating and reviewing systems

Making health systems more sustainable is part of a continuing journey that, importantly, includes evaluating our actions in a robust and efficient way at every step. If such evaluations take place at pre-defined intervals, they allow us to learn lessons and inform future actions that we may want or need to take. For the health sector, we can identify a number of crucial areas where monitoring, reviewing and evaluating what we are doing has the greatest benefits. We have covered these areas throughout this book. Figure 12.3 highlights again those topics that are particularly worth focusing on.

Can we get an overall sense of how we are doing so far? In Chapter 1 we talked of a 'crisis of compass' relating to the overall direction of the healthcare

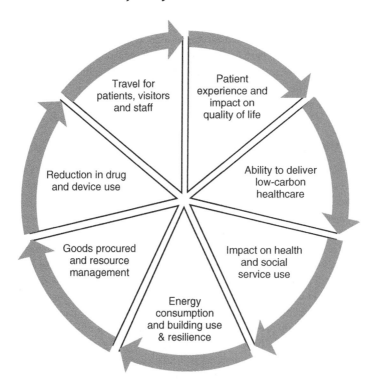

Figure 12.3 Evaluating and reviewing systems.

enterprise. While economic growth is the normal yardstick for the world's economies, in healthcare we chase the more elusive goal of good health, a subjective state rather than something we can easily measure. In 'greening the gaze', we add further complexity by bringing our planetary system into the equation. When we over-exploit natural resources to preserve human biological life 'at all costs', we undermine the whole system that sustains us. Fortunately, governments are starting to think about national success using measures other than *Gross Domestic Product (GDP)*, which, according to JF Kennedy, 'measures everything . . . except that which makes life worthwhile' [38]. For instance, the UK's *Office for National Statistics* was commissioned to measure the *happiness* of the UK population (76% of adults rated their life satisfaction with scores of seven or more out of ten) [39]. But again, focusing on happiness begs the question 'at what cost?'. The innovative *Happy Planet Index (HPI)* addresses this concern by combining the three variables of subjective life satisfaction, life expectancy and ecological footprint per capita. Conventionally, rich countries score averagely (for example, the UK ranked 74th and the US 114th out of 143 in 2009), while South and Central America do well, and sub-Saharan Africa comes out worst [40]. Perhaps this is the sort of sophisticated metric we need in healthcare as we engage in the fraught task of balancing individual patient expectations, the opportunities heralded by high-technology care and the need to live well together and sustainably?

Final thoughts

As we have demonstrated at the start of this book, our planet faces many serious crises. Globally, carbon dioxide emissions are rising rather than falling, and we are approaching, or surpassing, all the planetary boundaries discussed in Chapter 1. We have also identified strong reasons for health systems to show an interest in planetary health and to get actively involved in trying to mitigate our planetary crises – climate change in particular. Whilst we have many reasons to celebrate what modern healthcare has to offer, many health systems still have serious systemic flaws. A recurrent theme in this book has been the paradoxical idea that in the richer world we can create more health through less healthcare; healthcare that is superbly efficient, compassionate and that focuses on prevention, self-care and lower-carbon interventions.

In this chapter we have shown how we can come closer to these aims. Some may argue that this process will take too long, and that only some global calamity will trigger us into action. This is a depressing thought, yet it is possible that change can happen fast. For example, it is astonishing how quickly and efficiently the nations of the world can reconfigure their economies when they are under pressure, as was shown during the world wars of the twentieth century. Constraining as it might feel, legislation is likely to play a major role in achieving transition and transformation, ranging from local policies on the sourcing of hospital food to binding international laws and treaties for curbing greenhouse gas emissions. As with legislation on seat belts in vehicles and smoking in public places, change can also happen relatively fast in healthcare – and with less uproar and resistance than we may expect. Green technology is likely to play an important role, particularly in sectors such as geo-engineering, low-carbon energy and sustainable agriculture. Paradoxically, some major carbon-emitting countries such as China are at the leading edge: in 2010 China added a colossal 16 gigawatts of wind energy capacity, half the world's new wind-stock for that year and a hefty 64% increase on 2009 [41].

In the meantime we can all make positive contributions in our private lives, at work and as advocates for better policy. Some actions in our personal sphere are easy (shopping locally), money saving (switching off lights and equipment when not needed) and enjoyable (cycling instead of using the car). Others (like cutting back on air travel) may require short-term sacrifice and the sort of deeper motivations discussed in Chapter 3. We are hugely influenced by what is considered 'normal' in our culture (that holiday in the sun or snow, those electronic goods). But what we perceive as being normal can change surprisingly quickly. Once a critical mass is infected with a new idea or trend, it may start to spread like wildfire [42]. So there is real hope that our small gestures will do good in their own right but also contribute to a larger shift in attitudes. Global environmental change causes adverse effects on health right now and probably much more so in the future unless we, our generation, decide to act decisively. It is our choice to act, and it will be our legacy. This is also our opportunity.

References

1. Meadows, D.H. (2009) *Thinking in Systems: A Primer*. Routledge.
2. Marmot, M. (2007) Achieving health equity: from root causes to fair outcomes. *Lancet*, **370**, 1153–1163.
3. World Health Organization and Healthcare Without Harm (2009) Healthy hospitals, healthy planet, healthy people: Addressing climate change in healthcare settings [Internet]. http://www.who.int/globalchange/publications/healthcare_settings/en/index.html [accessed 2 August 2011].
4. NHS Sustainable Development – Unit Case studies [Internet]. http://www.sdu.nhs.uk/publications-resources/case-studies.aspx [accessed 28 October 2011].
5. International Council of Nurses (ICN) – Position Statements [Internet]. ttp://www.icn.ch/publications/position-statements/ [accessed 3 August 2011].
6. The World Federation of Public Health Associations (2001) GlobalClimateChange [Internet]. http://www.wfpha.org/tl_files/doc/resolutions/positionpapers/enrivonment/GlobalClimateChange.pdf [accessed 3 August 2011].
7. Centers for Disease Control and Prevention – Climate and Health Program (Homepage) [Internet]. http://www.cdc.gov/climatechange/ [accessed 3 August 2011].
8. Singh, S., Mushtaq, U., Holm-Hansen, C., Milan, D., Cheung, A. and Watts, N. (2011) The importance of climate change to health. *Lancet*, **378** (9785), 29–30.
9. Mazar, N. and Zhong, C.B. Do Green Products Make Us Better People? Psychological Science, 2010 21 (4), 494–498.
10. Health Care Without Harm (2011) HCWH Launches Global Environmental Health Agenda for Hospitals [Internet]. [http://www.noharm.org/global/news_hcwh/2011/oct/hcwh2011-10-13.php [accessed 3 November 2011].
11. Global Green and Healthy Hospitals Network [Internet]. http://www.greenhospitals.net/ [accessed 25 November 2011].
12. Health Care Without Harm (Home) [Internet]. http://www.noharm.org/ [accessed 5 August 2011].

13. NHS Sustainable Development Unit (2012) Sustainability in the NHS: Health Check 2012 [Internet]. http://www.sdu.nhs.uk/healthcheck2012 [accessed 21 February 2012].
14. Lorenzoni, I. and Pidgeon, N.F. (2006) Public Views on Climate Change: European and USA Perspectives. *Climatic Change*, **77** (1–2), 73–95.
15. NHS Sustainable Development Unit (2009) Fit for the Future [Internet]. http://www.sdu.nhs.uk/publications-resources/4/Fit-for-the-Future-/ [accessed 6 August 2011].
16. Harvard School of Public Health: Health Literacy Studies Web Site [Internet]. http://www.hsph.harvard.edu/healthliteracy/ [accessed 6 August 2011].
17. Health Literacy Group – Welcome to the Health Literacy Group website [Internet]. http://www.healthliteracy.org.uk/ [accessed 6 August 2011].
18. Self Care Forum (Home) [Internet]. http://www.selfcareforum.org/ [accessed 6 August 2011].
19. The Health Foundation (2011) Evidence: Helping people help themselves [Internet]. http://www.health.org.uk/publications/evidence-helping-people-help-themselves/ [accessed 27 February 2012].
20. Centre for Sustainable Healthcare (2011) Telephone clinics in the follow up of renal transplant recipients [Internet]. http://sustainablehealthcare.org.uk/green-nephrology/resources/2011/06/telephone-clinics-follow-renal-transplant-recipients [accessed 18 May 2012].
21. Health England – Publications [Internet]. http://www.healthengland.org/health_england_publications.htm [accessed 28 May 2012].
22. Blair, S.N., Kohl, III, H.W., Barlow, C.E., Paffenbarger, Jr, R.S., Gibbons, L.W. and Macera, C.A. (1995) Changes in physical fitness and all-cause mortality. A prospective study of healthy and unhealthy men. *Journal of the American Medical Association*, **273** (14), 1093–1098.
23. WHO (2004) World report on road traffic injury prevention [Internet]. http://www.who.int/violence_injury_prevention/publications/road_traffic/world_report/en/index.html [accessed 23 October 2011].
24. Battisti, D.S. and Naylor, R.L. (2009) Historical Warnings of Future Food Insecurity with Unprecedented Seasonal Heat. *Science*, **323** (5911), 240–244.
25. Frumkin, H., McMichael, A.J. and Hess, J.J. (eds) (2008) Climate Change and the Health of the Public. *American Journal of Preventive Medicine* (Theme issue), **35** (5), A1–A2, 401–538. [Internet: http://www.sciencedirect.com/science/journal/07493797/35/5] [accessed 31 July 2011].
26. BMJ – Fiona Godlee's carbon blog [Internet]. http://www.bmj.com/content/332/7554/suppl/DC1 [accessed 31 July 2011].
27. BMJ Group blogs – David Pencheon: Good general practice is sustainable general practice and vice versa [Internet]. http://blogs.bmj.com/bmj/2011/11/02/david-pencheon-good-general-practice-is-sustainable-general-practice-and-vice-versa/ [accessed 7 November 2011].
28. Madrid, P.A. and Grant, R. (2008) Meeting mental health needs following a natural disaster: Lessons from Hurricane Katrina. *Professional Psychology: Research and Practice*, **39** (1), 86–92.

29. Kovats, R.S. and Hajat, S. (2008) Heat Stress and Public Health: A Critical Review. *Annual Review of Public Health*, **29** (1), 41–55.
30. Leonardi, G. (2009) *How to prepare for the health effects of climate change. The health practitioner's guide to climate change*. Earthscan Ltd, London.
31. United Nations International Strategy for Disaster Reduction website [Internet]. http://www.unisdr.org/ [accessed 13 August 2011].
32. Environmental protection Agency – Climate Change Impacts and Adapting to Change [Internet]. http://www.epa.gov/climatechange/effects/adaptation.html [accessed 13 August 2011].
33. BMJ Group blogs – David Pencheon: Moral offset [Internet]. http://blogs .bmj.com/bmj/2010/10/04/david-pencheon-moral-offset/ [accessed 25 November 2011].
34. United Nations Environment Programme (UNEP) (1972) Rio Declaration on Environment and Development [Internet]. [http://www.unep.org/Documents .multilingual/Default.asp?DocumentID=78&ArticleID=1163 [accessed 11 December 2011].
35. NHS Sustainable Development Unit (2011) Route Map for Sustainable Health. NHS Sustainable Development Unit, Cambridge.
36. Hopkins, R. (2008) *The Transition Handbook: From Oil Dependency to Local Resilience*. Green Books, Totnes, UK.
37. Transition Edinburgh University – Research Database [Internet]. http://www .transitionedinburghuni.org.uk/projects/research/research-database/ [accessed 13 December 2011].
38. John F. Kennedy Presidential Library & Museum (1968) Remarks of Robert F. Kennedy at the University of Kansas, March 18, 1968 – [Internet]. http://www.jfklibrary.org/Research/Ready-Reference/RFK-Speeches/Remarks-of -Robert-F-Kennedy-at-the-University-of-Kansas-March-18-1968.aspx [accessed 27 May 2012].
39. Office for National Statistics (2011) Initial investigation into Subjective Well-being from the Opinions Survey [Internet].http://www.ons.gov.uk/ons/rel/wellbeing/ measuring-subjective-wellbeing-in-the-uk/investigation-of-subjective-well -being-data-from-the-ons-opinions-survey/initial-investigation-into-subjective -well-being-from-the-opinions-survey.html [accessed 27 May 2012].
40. Happy Planet Index (home) [Internet]. http://www.happyplanetindex.org/ [accessed 27 May 2012].
41. Global Wind Energy Council (GWEC) – PR China [Internet]. http://www .gwec.net/index.php?id=125 [accessed 29 May 2012].
42. Gladwell, M. (2002) *The Tipping Point: How Little Things Can Make a Big Difference*. Abacus, London.

Index

Note: Page numbers in *italics* refer to Figures; those in **bold** to Tables.

Sustainable Healthcare, First Edition. Knut Schroeder, Trevor Thompson, Kathleen Frith
and David Pencheon.
© 2013 John Wiley & Sons, Ltd. Published 2013 by John Wiley & Sons, Ltd.

Printed and bound by CPI Group (UK) Ltd, Croydon, CR0 4YY

09/10/2024

14571430-0002